TRANSITIONS TO ADULTHOOD

for Youth With Disabilities
Through an Occupational Therapy Lens

TRANSITIONS TO ADULTHOOD

for Youth With Disabilities
Through an Occupational Therapy Lens

Edited by

Debra Stewart, MSc, OT Reg (Ont)
Associate Professor
Occupational Therapy Program
School of Rehabilitation Science
McMaster University
Hamilton, Ontario, Canada

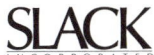

SLACK
INCORPORATED

ISBN: 978-1-61711-013-9

Instructors: *Transition to Adulthood for Youth With Disabilities Through an Occupational Therapy Lens, Instructor's Manual,* is also available from SLACK Incorporated. Don't miss this important companion to *Transition to Adulthood for Youth With Disabilities Through an Occupational Therapy Lens.* To obtain the *Instructor's Manual,* please visit http://www.efacultylounge.com.

Published by: SLACK Incorporated
                  6900 Grove Road
                  Thorofare, NJ 08086 USA
                  Telephone: 856-848-1000
                  Fax: 856-848-6091
                  www.Healio.com/books

Contact SLACK Incorporated for more information about other books in this field or about the availability of our books from distributors outside the United States.

Library of Congress Cataloging-in-Publication Data
Transitions to adulthood for youth with disabilities through an occupational therapy lens / [edited by] Debra Stewart.
    p. ; cm.
 Includes bibliographical references and index.
 ISBN 978-1-61711-013-9 (alk. paper)
 I. Stewart, Debra, 1954-
 [DNLM: 1. Child. 2. Disabled Persons--rehabilitation. 3. Adolescent. 4. Life Change Events. 5. Occupational Therapy. 6. Young Adult. WS 368]
 618.9289'165--dc23
                      2012024283

Printed in the United States of America.

Last digit is print number: 10   9   8   7   6   5   4   3   2   1

Dedication

To my parents,
who have provided constant support during my lifecourse.

Contents

Dedication .... *v*

Acknowledgments .... *ix*

About the Editor .... *xi*

Contributing Authors .... *xiii*

Introduction .... *xv*

Chapter 1   Transition to Adulthood for Youth With Disabilities:
Evidence to Support Occupational Therapy Practice 1
Debra Stewart, MSc, OT Reg (Ont)

Chapter 2   The McMaster Lens for Occupational Therapists: Linking
Theory to Practice 27
Mary Law, PhD, FCAOT, FCAHS

Chapter 3   Transitions From Parents' Home to Independent Living Arrangements
for Youth With Physical Disabilities... 47
*Andrea Morrison, BSc, OT Reg (Ont); Karen Margallo, MClSc (OT); and
Matt Freeman, MA*

Chapter 4   Community Participation Through Work Experience for Youth
With Developmental Disabilities 67
Linda Armour, BSc; Jan Burke-Gaffney; and Debra Stewart, MSc, OT Reg (Ont)

Chapter 5   Transition to Post-Secondary Education for Youth With Learning
Disabilities Using Assistive Technology 77
*Baljit Samrai, MSc, BSc, BHSc, OT Reg (Ont); Kim Carey, Hons B Kin, OT Reg (Ont);
and Christy Taberner, OT Reg (Ont)*

Chapter 6   Employment Transitions for Youth With Mental Health Issues 103
Sandra Moll, PhD, OT Reg (Ont) and Kevin Tregunno

Chapter 7   Socialization and Leisure Pursuits for Youth Living With Obesity
as the Result of a Complex Health Condition.. 123
Mary Forhan, PhD, OT Reg (Ont) and Grace Herron

Chapter 8   Future Directions in Practice and Research: Our Own Transitions....................... 135
Debra Stewart, MSc, OT Reg (Ont)

Financial Disclosures *153*

Index *155*

Acknowledgments

I have always been a "clinical" occupational therapist, and consider myself fortunate to still be working in a private practice with a great group of occupational therapists. But, I have also made my own transitions during my adult years into academic and research roles. I was supported and guided through these transitions by some incredible mentors—Mary Law, Sue Baptiste, and Cheryl Missiuna. I also want to acknowledge the ongoing support of the community of faculty and clinicians at McMaster University—the collaborative culture of our community inspired the development of this book.

My family has always been there for me—thanks for your support. My two "emerging adults" are a constant inspiration. A very special thank you to my daughter Trisha for her great photography and excellent PowerPoint skills.

This book has become an important part of my life journey. I made the decision to write this book instead of pursuing a PhD. The experience of writing and editing gave me the opportunity to work with a wonderful group of occupational therapists, community members, and the publishing staff at SLACK Incorporated. A special thanks to all of the authors of this book—you made it come alive. I appreciate all of your hard work and willingness to share your experiences. A big thank you to Tara Embrey for editing and formatting our work.

I can also say now that this book has been the best way for me to give back something to all of the people who have worked with me and taught me so much.

- » The young adults who first introduced me to the issues facing youth with disabilities during their transitions to adulthood—Danielle, Rob, Dulci, Annette, Josh, Todd, Doreen, Jennifer, and Paul

- » Sandra Sahagian Whalen, who partnered with me in the "early years" of our clinical research and the development of a peer mentorship program

- » The youth and their families who have shared their stories with me about their transition experiences and taught me about resilience and self-advocacy for full inclusion

- » Members of the Hamilton Family Network, who opened my eyes about citizenship and real community participation…"It's all about relationships!"

About the Editor

Debra Stewart, MSc, OT Reg (Ont), is an Associate Professor in the Occupational Therapy program in the School of Rehabilitation Science at McMaster University in Hamilton, Ontario, Canada. She is also a investigator at CanChild Centre for Childhood Disability Research, which is also at McMaster University. Her primary research interests include the transition to adulthood for youth with disabilities, and the use of the International Classification of Function Disability and Health from the World Health Organization. She has been the principal investigator for a number of research studies on the transition to adulthood including the development of best practice guidelines in Ontario; development and evaluation of a Youth KIT; and a Canadian study of the transitional tensions facing youth with disabilities.

Contributing Authors

Linda Armour, BSc, worked at the McMaster Hospital Chedoke Child and Family Centre in Hamilton, Ontario, Canada for 35 years. She presently works in family support at Community Living Hamilton. She was a Professional Associate at McMaster School of Rehabilitation Science, and currently is a board member of the Hamilton Family Network.

Jan Burke-Gaffney is a founder of the Hamilton Family Network, a parent-to-parent organization that seeks innovative, family-centered solutions by implementing strategies to support and strengthen families who have a member with a disability in Hamilton, Ontario, Canada. She is a professional associate in the School of Rehabilitation Science at McMaster University; co-investigator of the "Keeping It Together" (KIT) project with CanChild Centre for Childhood Disability Research at McMaster University; and past president of Family Alliance Ontario. Jan and her husband have 4 wonderful children who have provided them with the inspiration that guides their work to support the self-determination and inclusion of people with disabilities.

Kim Carey, Hons B Kin, OT Reg (Ont) has worked in the area of assistive technology for the past 6 years. She is affiliated with an expanded level augmentative and alternative communication clinic with the Ministry of Health and Long Term Care in Ontario. Her research interests include development of assistive technology strategies to promote independence in the home and school environment.

Mary Forhan, PhD, OT Reg (Ont) is an assistant clinical professor in the Occupational Therapy Program, School of Rehabilitation Science at McMaster University and an adjunct assistant professor, Department of Occupational Therapy, Faculty of Rehabilitation Medicine at the University of Alberta. She was a post-doctoral research fellow in the Department of Family Medicine at McMaster University at the time of writing this chapter. Her primary research interests are the participation in everyday living for persons with obesity and participation in primary and specialized care for the prevention and management of chronic health conditions.

Matt Freeman, MA is a PhD student in the Rehabilitation Science Program at McMaster University, Hamilton, Ontario, Canada. He has a masters degree in political science, and is interested in policy related to the transition to adulthood for youth with disabilities. Matt was a research assistant on several projects about the transition to adulthood including the development and evaluation of the Youth KIT, development of best practice guidelines in Ontario, and a Canada-wide study of the transitional tensions of youth with disabilities.

Grace Herron is a student at Brock University in St. Catharines, Ontario, Canada. She is majoring in child and youth studies and has a developing interest in linguistics. Post graduation she is considering speech language pathology as a career focus but is keeping in mind other options as well. She has volunteered at daycare facilities and elementary schools in her community, which has reinforced her desire to work with children.

Mary Law, PhD, FCAOT, FCAHS is a Professor in the School of Rehabilitation Science at McMaster University and an adjunct professor at La Trobe University in Melbourne, Australia. She holds the John and Margaret Lillie Chair in Childhood Disability Research. Mary is co-founder of CanChild Centre for Childhood Disability Research, a multidisciplinary research centre at McMaster University. Mary's research centers on evaluation of occupational therapy interventions with children, and the effect of environmental factors on the participation of children with disabilities in everyday occupations.

Karen Margallo, MClSc (OT) is an occupational therapist at the Children's Developmental Rehabilitation Programme (CDRP), an out-patient rehabilitation program at McMaster Children's Hospital, Hamilton, Ontario, Canada. Karen's clinical interests are in the practice area of pediatrics, in particular transition to adult living, spasticity management, and autism spectrum disorders. Her roles within CDRP include providing clinical services to children and youth with neurodevelopmental disabilities and/or functional issues, as well as Teen Transition Services. She is co-coordinator of the "Moving On" Teen Independence Program. Karen is also a Professional Associate with the School of Rehabilitation Sciences at McMaster University.

Sandra Moll, PhD, OT Reg (Ont) is an Assistant Professor in the Occupational Therapy program, School of Rehabilitation Science at McMaster University. She has over 10 years of clinical occupational therapy experience, primarily in the area of community mental health. Her primary research interests are in the area of mental health policy and practice, psychosocial disability, and work.

Andrea Morrison, BSc, OT Reg (Ont) is an occupational therapist at the Children's Developmental Rehabilitation Programme (CDRP), at Hamilton Health Sciences, McMaster Children's Hospital, Hamilton, Ontario, Canada. In her work with adolescents with physical and developmental disabilities, Andrea enjoys developing and facilitating community-based life skills programs and a youth advisory group that offers clients opportunity for peer networking and advocacy. Andrea is participating in clinical and research activities related to interventions that facilitate the transition of youth with chronic health conditions into adulthood. She is also a preceptor, tutor, and course co-coordinator with the Occupational Therapy program, School of Rehabilitation Science at McMaster University.

Baljit Samrai, MSc, BSc, BHSc, OT Reg (Ont) is involved with the Occupational Therapy Program at McMaster University as a part-time Assistant Clinical Professor. She has worked in the area of assistive technology for over 10 years. She is affiliated with an expanded level augmentative and alternative communication clinic with the Ministry of Health and Long Term Care in Ontario, Canada. In addition, Baljit has been involved in multiple research projects such as training protocols for speech recognition software and the use of the International Classification of Function Disability and Health from the World Health Organization.

Christy Taberner, OT Reg (Ont) is faculty in the Accessible Learning Services department at Mohawk College in Hamilton, Ontario, Canada. Christy is also an active member on the College's accessibility planning committee. Her primary research interests include transition planning for youth with disabilities entering post-secondary education and eHealth/mHealth solutions, which promote consumer engagement, empowerment, and health promotion.

Kevin Tregunno is a Recovery Support worker for an early intervention program at St Joseph's Healthcare in Hamilton, Ontario, Canada. He graduated from Mohawk College with a diploma in Recreation and Leisure services in 2002 and graduated with honors from the Psychosocial Rehabilitation certificate program in 2010. He went on to study addiction at McMaster University. He spends his spare time practicing mindfulness, writing poetry, spending quality time with his friends, and working toward an undergraduate degree.

Introduction

Two occupational therapists who work on the adolescent team at a children's rehabilitation program have heard from former clients who were discharged at age 19. These young adults have indicated that they are sitting at home (their parents' homes) with nothing much to do as they cannot get a job, and they don't know what to do. The occupational therapists get approval to run a series of focus groups in the summer about "vocational readiness" to find out what they could be doing to assist their clients in preparing for future adult roles in the workforce. They invite seven former clients, ages 20 to 25, to be participants. At the first session, the participants agree that employment is only one transition that they are having difficulty with. They make it clear that the occupational therapists, and the adolescent team, have to look beyond vocational readiness and work to address the whole picture of transitions to adult life. The year was 1990.

The scenario described above was not an isolated one—there were many similar situations in different settings and countries that emerged in the 1980s and into the 1990s. Back then, there was some literature that described the experiences of youth with lifelong (also referred to in the literature as "congenital" or "chronic") disabilities as they entered the adult world. These youth had grown up in their own community, living at home with their families and attending public schools, many integrated into mainstream education. They were therefore expecting to enter into the mainstream of adult society, and they had dreams and aspirations that were similar to their peers without disabilities—to pursue further education, to find a job, to enter into adult relationships, and to move out of their parents' homes someday. But, when these youth with disabilities graduated from high school and were too old for pediatric services, reality hit and they were feeling frustrated, disappointed, and alone.

Why was this happening? Medical advancements in the 1960s and 1970s increased the survival rates of infants born with different types of impairments. As children, they continued to develop into "healthy" adolescents with the support of medical, rehabilitation, and social services. At the same time, institutions were being closed and these children and youth were living in their own communities. Public education systems were changing to include and accommodate children and youth with exceptionalities. Other systems and services were responding to the increasing number of youth with disabilities in the 1970s and 1980s by establishing adolescent programs in communities (Rusch, Destefano, Chadsey-Rusch, Phelps, & Szymanski, 1992).

Thus, a new reality was emerging. Children with different types of lifelong disabilities (e.g., physical, medical, developmental, emotional, learning, and social) became adolescents who had longer life expectancies and wanted to remain in their communities as adults. These youth and their families had worked hard and advocated to be integrated and included in community life, and they were expecting the same as they entered adult society. In the past, however, there had been no or little planning to prepare them for living in their own communities as adults, and the various adult systems were not ready for them.

As this new reality emerged, youth with disabilities and their families voiced their concerns and frustrations. And people within different systems and services began to listen and respond. Governments commissioned studies to learn more about the current status of youth with disabilities. For example, in the United States, the first National Education Longitudinal Study (Institute of Education Sciences [IES], 1988) gathered data about transitions experienced by students, including those with special needs, starting in grade eight, through high school, and into postsecondary institutions or the work force. And in 1991, the first National Longitudinal Survey of Youth in Transition (NLTS) (Wagner et al., 1991) started to study the experiences and outcomes of students with special education needs. Education systems were responding with policy changes that addressed the needs of students with special needs by implementing "transition plans" as part of the individualized education plans for all students with exceptionalities ages 14 and older (Leucking & Wittenburg, 2009). In health and social systems, research was conducted to learn about the needs of adolescent clients in order to establish client-centered and developmentally appropriate services and supports (Parmenter & Knox, 1991; Wells, Sandefur, & Hogan, 2003). In 1993, the Society for Adolescent Medicine published a position paper about the transition from pediatric to adult health care services for adolescents with chronic conditions (Blum et al., 1993). These efforts in the systems in which youth with disabilities receive services and supports have increased in the past two decades and can be found in many countries.

Why is this important now? Statistics from recent census surveys in the United States report that almost 10% of persons under the age of 25 have some form of disability (Steinmetz, 2006). Demographic data from research about adolescents and young adults indicates that the proportion of young people with lifelong/chronic conditions increases with age, to peak at about 17% for ages 12 to 17 years (Wood, Reiss, Ferris, Edwards, & Merrick, 2010). Data from other countries are not as precise for the adolescent and young adult years, but many experts indicate that a growing number of youth with lifelong disabilities are reaching adulthood each year. There is also evidence that unemployment rate for young adults with disabilities is higher than those with no disabilities (Human Resources Social Development Canada, 2002; Janus, 2009; Wagner, Newman, Cameto, & Levine, 2005). We, therefore, need to continue to build on the efforts and progress made to date.

We have made progress in the past few decades. Our understanding about the transitions to adulthood for youth with disabilities has evolved from a focus on "event markers," such as getting a job and getting married, to a continuous developmental process that involves the interaction of person and environment over time (Gorter, Stewart, & Woodbury-Smith, 2011). The title of this book also reflects current views that the process involves multiple transitions in different domains, such as employment, education, living arrangements, community participation, socialization, and leisure. We also have a growing body of evidence about the experiences, factors, and outcomes of these transitions for youth with different disabilities and some examples of evidence-based programs in different sectors. Recent studies have shown that the efforts of governments and services are having a modest, positive influence on the transition outcomes for youth with disabilities. The second wave of the National Longitudinal Transition Study (NLTS-II) in 2005 found that the unemployment rate for an aggregate sample of all youth with disabilities had improved by approximately 9% (Wagner et al., 2005). However, certain populations of youth with disabilities had much lower employment rates, including those with intellectual or significant/complex disabilities. Studies from other countries have also shown some improvements in services and supports for youth with disabilities (Wood et al., 2010).

We still, however, have a long way to go, and if we want to continue to move forward in a positive direction, we all need to take responsibility to be evidence based and proactive in our practice. And "we" includes occupational therapists. There is relatively little evidence about occupational therapy practice in the literature on adult transitions for youth with disabilities. Descriptive articles written by a few occupational therapists back in the 1980s and 1990s identified the need for our services and suggested ways for us to get involved (Brollier, Shepherd, & Markley, 1994; Clark, Mack, & Pennington, 1989; Spencer, 1996). Today, most of the occupational therapy literature on this topic is still primarily descriptive in nature, although there are some recent studies upon which we can build, and this book presents the evidence.

The main purpose of this book is to provide occupational therapy students and clinicians with the tools they need to contribute actively to developing the services, supports, and thinking needed for positive, successful adult transitions for youth with lifelong disabilities. These tools include current evidence to inform our practice, the framework of an occupational therapy lens to guide professional reasoning, and examples of application of this lens with different occupations, settings, and youth populations. The Instructor's Manual for this book provides additional information on tools for thinking and learning.

There are a few important points to keep in mind for readers of this book. It is recommended that you start with the first two chapters of the book. Chapter 1 presents a comprehensive overview of research evidence, but it also identifies the need for theoretical evidence at the current stage of knowledge. Chapter 2 describes The McMaster Lens for Occupational Therapists (Salvatori et al., 2006) as a tool to connect theory with practice and to demonstrate how to use available evidence to inform practice decisions. The next five chapters can be read in any order. They are organized by the types of transition domains (or occupations through an occupational therapy lens) that include self-care (independent living and community management), productivity (education and employment), and leisure/socialization. Each chapter focuses on one domain/occupation in relation to one youth population. The population approach was purposefully taken, versus a focus on specific conditions or diagnoses, as recent evidence indicates that the issues, supports, and strategies for transitions to adulthood are similar for youth with different conditions and diagnoses, which acknowledges that the diagnosis of the young person should not be the focus of occupational therapy reasoning and practice. Each chapter starts with a scenario of an individual, to promote a client-centered and individualized approach to practice, but the clinical reasoning of the therapists and the theories, models, and strategies presented can be generalized to many other practice situations with different youth populations.

The term *evidence* in this book includes more than research or literature. Therapists use multiple forms of evidence to make decisions, including different types of research (quantitative, qualitative), their own practice experiences and professional context, and the perspectives, values, and experiences of clients and families (Law, Pollock, & Stewart, 2004; Palisano, 2010). All of these forms of evidence are considered important and relevant in this book. Furthermore, theoretical evidence, in the form of models and theories that have been evaluated and critiqued, is included to demonstrate its importance in professional reasoning and decision making.

All of the authors in this book are from one community. This was also a purposeful decision. The community of the occupational therapy program at McMaster University in Hamilton, Ontario, Canada is renowned for evidence-based and client-centered practice. The strong relationship between the university and the clinical community fosters a collaborative network of occupational therapists. Those of us who work with children and youth with disabilities draw upon the evidence and support provided by CanChild Centre for Childhood Disability Research (see www.canchild.ca). This book is not about the McMaster community specifically. Rather, it uses this community to demonstrate how occupational therapists from local academic and clinical settings can collaborate with youth and their families and other services and systems to foster positive outcomes. This book is intended to provide evidence, a framework, and application examples for occupational therapists who believe in using a client-centered, evidence-based community approach to address the transitions to adulthood for youth with lifelong disabilities.

References

Blum, R. W., Garell, D., Hodgman, C. H., Jorissen, T. W., Okinow, N. A., Orr, D. P., & Slap, G. B. (1993). Transition from child-centred to adult health-care systems for adolescents with chronic conditions. A position paper of the Society for Adolescent Medicine. *Journal of Adolescent Health, 14*(7), 570-576.

Brollier, C., Shepherd, J., & Markley, K. F. (1994). Transition from school to community living. *American Journal of Occupational Therapy, 48*(4), 346-353.

Clark, F. A., Mack, W., & Pennington, V. (1989). Transition needs assessment of severely disabled high school students and their parents and teachers. *Occupational Therapy Journal of Research, 8*(6), 323-344.

Gorter, J. W., Stewart, D., & Woodbury-Smith, M. (2011). Youth in transition: Care, health, and development. *Child: Care, Health, and Development, 37*(6), 757-763.

Human Resources Social Development Canada (HRSDC) (2002). *Advancing the inclusion of people with disabilities.* Otttawa, Ontario, Canada: Government of Canada.

Institute of Educational Sciences (IES). (1988). *National Education Longitudinal Survey (NELS:88).* Retrieved from http://nces.ed.gov/surveys/nels88

Janus, A. L. (2009). Disability and the transition to adulthood. *Social Forces, 88* (1), 99-120.

Law, M., Pollock, N., & Stewart, D. (2004). Evidence-based occupational therapy: Concepts and strategies. *New Zealand Journal of Occupational Therapy, 51*(1), 14-22.

Luecking, R. G., & Wittenburg, D. (2009). Providing supports to youth with disabilities transitioning to adulthood: Case descriptions from the youth transition demonstration. *Journal of Vocational Rehabilitation, 30*(3), 241-251.

Palisano, R. J. (2010). Practice knowledge: The forgotten aspect of evidence-based practice. *Physical and Occupational Therapy in Pediatrics, 30*(4), 261-263.

Parmenter, T. R., & Knox, M. (1991). The post-school experiences of young people with a disabiliy. *International Journal of Rehabilitation Research, 14*(4), 281-291.

Rusch, F. R., Destefano, L., Chadsey-Rusch, J., Phelps L. A., & Szymanski, E. (Eds.). (1992). *Transition from school to adult life.* Pacific Grove, CA: Brooks/Cole Publishing Co.

Salvatori, P., Jung, B., Missiuna, C., Stewart, D., Law, M., & Wilkins, S. (2006). *The McMaster lens for occupational therapists.* Hamilton, Ontario, Canada: McMaster University.

Spencer, K. (1996). Transition services: From school to adult life. In J. Case-Smith, A. S. Allen, & P. N. Pratt (Eds.), *Occupational therapy for children* (pp. 808-822). St. Louis, MO: Mosby Year Book Inc.

Steinmetz, E. (2006). *Americans with disabilities.* Washington, DC: US Census Bureau.

Wagner, M., Newman, L., Cameto, R., & Levine, P. (2005). *National Longitudinal Transition Study 2: Changes over time in the early postschool outcomes of youth with disabilities.* Menlo Park, CA: SRI International.

Wagner, M., Newman, L., D'Amico, R., Jay, E.D., Butler-Nalin, P., Marder, C., Cox, R. (1991). *Youth with disabilities: How are they doing? The first comprehensive report from the national longitudinal transition study.* Menlo Park, CA: SRI International.

Wells, T., Sandefur, G. D., & Hogan, D. P. (2003). What happens after the high school years among young persons with disabilities? *Social Forces, 82*(2), 803-832.

Wood, D., Reiss, J. G., Ferris, M. E., Edwards, L. R., & Merrick, J. (2010). Transition from pediatric to adult care. *International Journal of Child and Adult Health, 3*(4), 445-447.

1

Transitions to Adulthood for Youth With Disabilities

Evidence to Support

Occupational Therapy Practice

Debra Stewart, MSc, OT Reg (Ont)

> James is 21 years old and lives at home with his parents and two siblings. He enjoys physical activity and socializing with other people. He has physical and developmental disabilities, and requires assistance or supervision for most activities. James is in a "life skills" class at his local high school, with two special education teachers and several teaching assistants for support. James is integrated for some classes, including music and physical education. He participates in a swim program every week and other recreational activities, such as bowling, as part of the school curriculum.
>
> School staff developed a transition plan with James and his mother that focused on exploring employment options. After he graduated from high school, he participated in a supported employment program for adults in his community on a part-time basis. James' mother is pleased that he has a program to go to during the day that is very different from high school. He does not have the same opportunities or supports to participate in community recreational activities as an adult. As a result, his parents are taking him swimming and bowling on their own, as they feel they are important activities for him. They are advocating for some inclusive recreational programs in the community that fit with his physical, social, and recreational assets and interests.

A developmental transition represents change and growth for any individual. The traditional views of development would describe transition as a change from one developmental stage to another (e.g., from adolescence to adulthood). Current theories and models about development view transition as a dynamic and interactional process between person and environment (Lerner, 2002). A developmental transition is part of a person's natural lifecourse, and represents a time of significant change and adaptation within the person and his or her environment. Many transitions occur in an individual's life journey, and they are associated with different challenges and opportunities, given the changes that are taking place.

Stewart, D. (Ed.)
Transitions to Adulthood for Youth With Disabilities
Through an Occupational Therapy Lens (pp. 1-26).
© 2013 SLACK Incorporated

The transition to adulthood can therefore be viewed as a dynamic process in which the trajectory of an individual's life journey shifts as the relationships between person and environment change. An occupational therapy view of this transition would expand upon this to include interactions between person, environment, and occupation. As an individual's roles and occupations within home, school, community, and even societal environments evolve, developmental expectations focus more on independence and responsibility. Significant environmental change occurs for all youth when they graduate from the education system of their adolescence and/or move out of the parental home.

For youth with lifelong or chronic disabilities, the process of transition from adolescence to adulthood is similar to typical youth in many ways—they too graduate from high school, and most have a desire to find work and move out of their parents' home at some point (Stewart et al., 2008). Research on the process and outcomes of this transition for youth with lifelong disabilities has identified numerous additional challenges as most face significant changes, such as discharge from pediatric health and social systems, and loss of community supports.

If occupational therapists are to provide evidence-based and client-centered services to youth with disabilities, we need to be aware of the current evidence about transitions to adulthood for youth with disabilities. As health professionals, our clinical reasoning must also be guided by current and relevant models and theories. This chapter will review the current evidence from both research and theoretical perspectives. The research evidence is reviewed first and is framed by the unique lens of occupational therapy that addresses person, environment, and occupation in an interactional way. The subheadings are the following:

≫ Person (P)—Evidence about the transition experiences and needs of youth with different types of lifelong/chronic conditions.

≫ Environment (E)—Including physical, social, cultural, and institutional/system environments. This will focus on evidence about environmental supports and barriers.

≫ Occupation (O)—Evidence about the different domains of transition, such as education, employment, independent living, and socialization.

≫ Evidence about PEO interactions that enable an individual's occupational performance and participation in daily life. This section will describe recent interactional approaches that address the complexity of the transition process.

Finally, research evidence about the effectiveness of current transition models of practice will be reviewed, along with evidence about occupational therapy services for this population.

Following the review of the research evidence, theoretical perspectives about the transition to adulthood will be presented. Theory is important to address when there is limited research evidence to support practice, and this chapter will show that this is the current state facing service providers in the area of transitions to adulthood for youth with disabilities. Occupational therapists, therefore, need to draw upon a combination of evidence from both research and theoretical perspectives to guide our clinical reasoning.

Research Evidence

There has been a dramatic increase in published literature about transition to adulthood for youth with disabilities in the past few decades. Table 1-1 illustrates the evolving nature of research as our knowledge about this topic has changed over time.

Research in the 1980s and 1990s brought attention to the issue, as poor outcomes in areas of employment, education, and living arrangements were identified in studies about youth with disabilities (Blackorby & Wagner, 1996; Levine & Nourse, 1998). Research then emerged about the experiences and needs of youth with different types of disabilities during this transition (Frank

Table 1-1.	
Research on Transitions to Adulthood	
No knowledge (1980s)	Descriptive and observational studies
Knowledge about the "problem"	Needs surveys and follow-up studies
Knowledge about the different "variables" (early 2000s)	Qualitative and cross-sectional studies about person-environment factors and outcomes
The complexity of the situation; finding a solution (current)	Demonstration/pilot studies Development of outcome measures Collaborative knowledge translation and mobilization projects
Different models (solutions) for different groups and communities (future)	Large, prospective, longitudinal studies using reliable, valid outcome measures

& Sitlington, 2000; Stewart, Law, Rosenbaum, & Willms, 2001). Other research explored the factors that influence the transition process, and this knowledge has influenced the development of "best practice" position papers and guidelines (Stewart et al., 2009). Recent literature is reporting evidence on models of practice that are building on the work from the past 20 to 30 years. It would be impossible to review all of the research about the transition to adulthood for youth with disabilities in this chapter. To inform and support evidence-based practice by occupational therapists in the current practice context, the research evidence that has been published since the year 2000 will be summarized using a PEO framework.

Evidence About "Person" Components

Literature reviews (Beresford, 2004; Reinehr, Dobe, Winkel, Schaefer, & Hoffmann, 2010; Seltzer, Shattuck, Abbeduto, & Greenberg, 2004; Stewart, Stavness, King, Antle, & Law, 2006) and findings from national longitudinal studies (Armstrong, Dedrick, & Greenbaum, 2003; Berzin, 2010; Hollar, 2005; Wagner, Newman, Cameto, & Levine, 2005; Wagner, Newman, Cameto, Levine, & Garza, 2006) provide current best evidence about personal factors that can influence the transition process. Other articles that focus on one population of youth or one study provide additional evidence. Personal factors are subdivided into positive factors that facilitate the transition process and risk factors or barriers to transition.

Personal Supports/Facilitators

Personal support factors, or facilitators, that have been identified in recent research about youth with disabilities in transition to adulthood include the following:

> Effective coping strategies, active engagement, perseverance, and goal setting (Learning Disabilities Association of Canada [LDAC], 2007; Stewart et al., 2008).

> Emotional intelligence; internal control and adaptive behavior; self-advocacy; disclosure skills; and knowledge about one's condition, rights, and future options (Baltodano, Mathur, & Rutherford, 2005; Blacher, 2001; Kerka, 2002).

> Literacy level and language skills and strong social and communication skills (Alpern & Zager, 2007; Kirby, Sugden, Beveridge, & Edwards, 2008; LDAC, 2007).

> Believing in oneself and having spiritual beliefs (King, Brown, & Smith, 2003; King, Cathers, Miller Polgar, MacKinnon, & Havens, 2000).

Self-determination has been identified in the literature as both a critical personal factor and a subjective outcome of adult transitions (Field & Hoffman, 2002; Lehman, Clark, Bullis,

Rinkin, & Castellanos, 2002; Powers, 2001; Stewart et al., 2008; Turnbull & Turnbull, 2006). Self-determination status has been linked to positive leisure, employment, and independent living outcomes (Martorell, Guteirrez-Rechacha, Pereda, & Ayuso-Mateos, 2008; McGuire & McDonnell, 2008; Wehmeyer & Palmer, 2003). The concept of self-determination has been studied extensively in the past two decades, most notably in the education system by Wehmeyer and colleagues (Wehmeyer, 2005; Wehmeyer, Abery, Mithaug, & Stancliffe, 2003). Self-determination refers to self-directed actions (versus actions that are caused or directed by others) and includes characteristics of autonomy, self-regulation, initiation, empowerment, and self-realization (Wehmeyer, 2005; Wehmeyer et al., 2003; Williams-Diehm, Wehmeyer, Palmer, Soukup, & Garner, 2008). The term *volitional behavior* has been used to describe self-determination, to highlight that a self-determined person is acting based on his or her own will, with conscious intention (Williams-Diehm et al., 2008). This fits closely with the concept of volition in Kielhofner's Model of Human Occupation (Kielhofner, 2008), which refers to the process whereby people choose the activities in which they are motivated to participate.

Studies about self-determination have found that this personal factor can have a strong influence on positive transition outcomes for youth with different types of disabilities (Algozzine, Browder, Karvonen, Test, & Wood, 2001; Wehmeyer & Palmer, 2003). An individual's self-determination can be influenced by his or her personal adaptive abilities as well as environmental opportunities to make choices and pursue his or her interests (Carter, Trainor, Owens, Sweden, & Sun, 2010). This evidence suggests that self-determination deserves a great deal of attention by occupational therapists and other professionals working with youth with disabilities.

Personal Risk Factors/Barriers

Several articles identify a person's condition or impairment to be a risk factor, such as physical, mental, behavioral, sensory, developmental, and/or learning disabilities (Baltodano et al., 2005; Binks, Barden, Burke, & Young, 2007; Cameto, Levine, & Wagner, 2004; LDAC, 2007; Vander Stoep, Weiss, McKnight, Beresford, & Cohen, 2002). Statistical evidence indicates that the type of disability can affect the process and outcomes of adult transitions (Caton & Kagan, 2007; Van Naarden Braun, Yeargin-Allsopp, & Lollar, 2006; Wells, Sandefur, & Hogan, 2003). Research articles that focus on one specific population of youth provide evidence about the type of impairment/condition as a factor influencing youth development. For example, Seltzer et al. (2004) concluded in a literature review about youth with autism spectrum disorder that Intelligence Quotient was the best predictor of adolescent or adult outcomes, although there was considerable variance in outcomes. Youth with mental illness/emotional challenges were found to have more risk-taking behaviors (Altshuler, Mackelprang, & Baker, 2008), and the proportion of these youth who completed high school was negatively influenced by the severity of the psychiatric illness (Vander Stoep et al., 2002).

Some research articles about youth with physical and developmental challenges also found comorbidities, or the presence of other conditions, to be an important influence in developmental processes (Horsman, Suto, Dudgeon, & Harris, 2010; Lounds, Seltzer, Greenberg, & Shattuck, 2007). In the most recent National Longitudinal Transition Study (NLTS-2), youth with multiple diagnoses or conditions were less likely to be employed than youth with other diagnoses, but those with higher social skills ratings were more likely to be employed (Wagner et al., 2005; Wagner et al., 2006). Some articles also report increased risk of negative outcomes, such as unemployment and health problems, with a high level of severity of disability (Bowe, 2003; Canadian National Institute for the Blind [CNIB], 2002; Caton & Kagan, 2007; Community Living Research Project, 2006; Wong, 2004).

Some authors, however, caution that disability is only one factor in the complex processes of development and transition (Burchardt, 2004; Gorter, Stewart, & Woodbury-Smith, 2011). Numerous other personal characteristics have been cited in the literature as risk factors for youth:

» Literature about Aboriginal, Hispanic, and African-American youth with disabilities speaks to the "double jeopardy" risk factors of disability and ethnicity (Blacher, 2001; Blackstock, Bruyere, & Moreau, 2006; Blue-Banning, Turnbull, & Pereira, 2002). There is statistical evidence that these young people have much poorer outcomes in all domains (Cameto et al., 2004), although a recent study in the United States (Van Naarden Braun et al., 2006) found that when researchers controlled for impairment, no demographic variables, including ethnicity and gender, were significant predictors of a successful transition outcome.

» Some research has found that there are significant differences in transition outcomes between men and women with disabilities (Berge, Patterson, Goetz, & Milla, 2007; Jonikas, Laris, & Cook, 2003). For example, Powers et al. (2008) found that females with impairments were lagging behind their male peers in terms of employment. However, there appear to be multiple interactions occurring with educational attainment, family background, and other personal factors.

» One review article noted that youth with low expectations and aspirations can have a more difficult transition (Beresford, 2004). The author also noted that youth who do not communicate through verbal speech are most vulnerable to problems with adult relationships and employment.

» Two studies of youth with orthopedic/physical disabilities found that personal risk factors for this population were pain, nutrition, sleep quality, cognitive functioning, and mobility status (Bartlett, Hanna, Avery, Stevenson, & Galuppi, 2010; Wright, Tancredi, Yundt, & Larin, 2006).

» Using data from the National Education Longitudinal Study (NELS: 88), Hollar (2005) found that substance abuse was higher for youth with disabilities compared to their peer group. Youth with learning, emotional, and multiple conditions appeared to be at the greatest risk for drug abuse.

All of these findings about personal characteristics were similar to those reported by Berzin (2010), who analyzed data from the National Longitudinal Survey of Youth and found that personal risk factors included intellectual ability, use of drugs, criminal activity, pregnancy, lack of personal agency, and a negative future outlook.

Evidence About "Environment" Components

Very few published articles focus solely on environmental barriers and/or supports, but the influence (both positive and negative) of environmental factors is embedded in recent literature about transitions to adulthood for youth with disabilities. The primary physical, social, and cultural environmental factors described in the literature are presented in this chapter. Table 1-2 organizes the various environmental factors into supports and barriers, as reported in the literature.

Physical Environment

Physical environment factors were identified in several review articles and longitudinal studies that focused primarily on youth with physical and developmental disabilities. Barriers included lack of physical access to buildings or transportation, while environmental supports included equipment and technology and physical adaptations within schools and workplaces (Colver, Dickinson, & SPARCLE group, 2010; Shikako-Thomas, Majnemer, Law, & Lach, 2008; Stewart et al., 2006). Technology, such as augmentative communication, can be a great support if used appropriately (Mull & Sitlington, 2003). Transportation options for youth and young adults with disabilities also greatly influences their ability to participate in community activities (Stewart et al., 2009).

Table 1-2. Environmental Factors That Influence Transitions to Adulthood for Youth With Disabilities—As Identified in the Literature	
Factors Identified as Supports	**Factors Identified as Barriers**
Physical Environment	
Access to all buildings, services, programs, transportation	Inaccessible buildings
Accessible public buses and trains	Restricted transportation options and schedules for persons with disabilities
Physical adaptations in schools and workplaces	"Special" equipment can be too costly
Social Environment	
Knowledge of options available by families and support staff	Lack of knowledge and understanding by service providers, educators, parents, and community members and needs of youth in transition
Positive peer relationships and supports	Bullying and staring by peers
Adult mentors/navigators in the community	Parents' (and others') low expectations for the future
Parents advocating for youth's participation, etc.	Lack of advocacy supports
Parents able to drive youth to activities	Low socioeconomic status of family; poverty
Cultural Environment	
Beliefs about inclusion and full participation for persons with disabilities	Stigma and discriminatory beliefs about persons with disabilities
Institutional Environment (Services, Systems, Government)	
Seamless transfer to adult services	Lack of availability of adult services
Transition coordinator to support the transfer between service systems	Lack of continuity between pediatric and adult services
Government financial aids and supports; adequate insurance coverage	Underfunding of services
Services focus on autonomy of youth	Services that foster dependency of youth
Community supports such as housing options and recreation programs	Lack of housing options for persons with disabilities
Accessible and usable information about transition and options for the future	Lack of information about "what's next?" and "what's out there?"
Policies and legislation that support persons with disabilities	Lack of government mandates/laws at different levels to support persons with disabilities
Temporal Environment	
Inclusive experiences in school and community through childhood and adolescence	Lack of opportunities, experiences, and choices in childhood and adolescence
Virtual Environment	
Technology, such as augmentative communication equipment	Technology being outdated or not available

> Susan is 24 years old and living at home with her mother and young brother. She has spina bifida and hydrocephalus and uses a manual wheelchair for mobility. Susan's future plans include paid employment. She is interested in working in an office environment as a receptionist and is taking college courses to upgrade her skills. She attends a college that is accessible and has supports for students with special needs, but it is in a different county than the one she lives in. The transportation system for people with disabilities does not cross county borders, so her mother must drive her every day. Susan knows that she also needs work experience and is doing some volunteer work. She is finding that many of the work settings are not physically accessible. She is concerned that she will have the skills needed for an office job, but will be unable to find a "user-friendly" work setting.

Social Environment

Many factors in the social environments of youth with disabilities have been identified in recent studies. The environment of the family can pose barriers, such as low socioeconomic status (SES). However, one study found that SES had a smaller impact on youth with disabilities than those with no disabilities (Wells et al., 2003). Other family factors that can act as either supports or barriers include parents' expectations for the future (Chambers, Hughes, & Carter, 2004), agreement with their youth on the importance of achieving adult goals (Powers, Geenen, & Powers, 2009), and their level of knowledge and information to help their young adult (LDAC, 2007). In qualitative studies, parents of youth with disabilities were found to be more pessimistic about the future than parents of students without disabilities (Magill-Evans, Wiart, Darrah, & Kratochvil, 2005). Some parents also experience more challenges with role changes and get frustrated trying to access appropriate services (Jivanjee, Kruzich, & Gordon, 2009). Recent studies indicate that parents benefit from being actively involved in transition planning, as they can then offer more help to their child in making decisions and planning for the future (Goupil, Tassé, Garcin, & Doré, 2002).

The level of knowledge about options and understanding of disability-related needs of youth by service providers, educators, and community members also affects a young person's transition process (Hitchings et al., 2001). Negative attitudes, such as low expectations and stereotyping, can lead to a lack of opportunities, choices, and experiences during the adolescent years, which can have a profound impact on adult outcomes (Foster & MacLeod, 2004). Stigma and discrimination have been identified by youth with disabilities in several recent studies (Shikako-Thomas et al., 2008; Stewart et al., 2006). On the other hand, positive attitudes and supports by adults have been shown to promote a positive trajectory (Stewart et al., 2008).

Friendships and peer supports have been viewed as positive factors influencing transitions to adulthood (Beresford, 2004; Kerka, 2002; Shikako-Thomas et al., 2008; Stewart et al., 2006). Peer mentorship has been viewed by youth with different types of disabilities to be an important influence as they make transitions to the adult world (Beresford, 2004; Stewart et al., 2001), as illustrated in Figure 1-1. Peer networks and mentoring relationships have been shown to provide positive support to youth and parents in accessing opportunities and experiences (Foster & MacLeod, 2004; Grove & Giraud-Saunders, 2003; Stewart et al., 2006). For example, an evaluation of a peer mentorship program for youth with physical disabilities demonstrated positive benefits for both mentors and mentees (Stewart, 2003). The program involved young adults with disabilities, ages 19 to 29 years old, being trained as mentors for young teenagers with disabilities (called *mentees*). Qualitative interviews with mentors, mentees, and parents at the end of the first year of the program showed that the younger mentee appreciated spending time with someone who had "been there, done that" (p. 201), which reduced his or her feelings of being alone. All participants in the program reported an increased sense of exploration and risk taking to try new activities (Stewart, 2003).

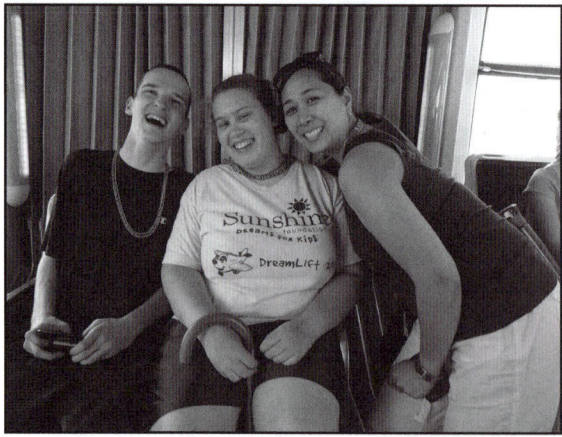

Figure 1-1. Youth with disabilities can provide peer support and mentorship.

Cultural Environment

The cultural environment is defined in the Occupational Therapy Practice Framework (American Occupation Therapy Association [AOTA], 2008) as the "customs, beliefs, activity patterns, behavior standards, and expectations accepted by the society of which the client is a member" (p. 645). This environment category includes political aspects and other systems in a society. Numerous barriers and supports have been identified within the culture of *services and systems*. Barriers include a lack of continuity from pediatrics to adult services (Committee on Disability in America, 2007; Davis & Sondheimer, 2005; Rapley & Davidson, 2010; Reiss, Gibson & Walker, 2005), lack of access to services, under funding of services, and lack of individualized and flexible service options (Darrah, Magill-Evans, & Galambos, 2010). The narrow focus of some services has also been identified as a barrier, for example, school systems that focus more on preparation for post-secondary education instead of addressing the lifecourse needs of youth in all domains of transition (Bowe, 2003). Within the education system, the influence of segregation versus integration/inclusion has been debated (Hetherington et al., 2010; Saigal et al., 2006), as well as the challenges involved in transferring from one school system, such as high school, to another, such as post-secondary education (Jivanjeet et al., 2009). In the health care system, some transition programs still focus exclusively on a youth's medical/health condition (Gorter et al., 2011) and ignore other aspects of a youth's life.

Supports within services and systems have also been identified in some studies. Supportive community-based systems include a range of options for attendant care and housing for young adults with different levels of support needs (Stewart et al., 2009). Service supports include useful information about disabilities, the transition process, and options for the future, to help a young person make informed decisions (Lehman et al., 2002).

Governments, with their associated policies and legislation, are large systems that can have a significant impact on the transition process for all youth with disabilities. A recent review of the transition literature found that most articles about legislation and policies come from North America (United States and Canada) and Europe (Germany and United Kingdom) (Kraus de Camargo, 2011).

Policy that is related to youth with disabilities in transition to adulthood falls into different types and systems of impact. At the broadest level of policy impact is overarching legislation about the rights of all persons with disabilities. The best-known legislation of this kind is the Americans with Disabilities Act (ADA) (P.L. 110-325). In Canada, the Charter of Rights and Freedoms addresses persons with disabilities, as does similar legislation in the United Kingdom and Australia.

The United States and the United Kingdom have national legislation that is intended to directly influence transition practices within specific systems. In the United Kingdom, the Autism Act (2009) mandates services for adults with autism spectrum disorder, in an attempt to address the poor transition outcomes of this population (McConachie, 2011). In the United States, the Individuals with Disabilities Education Improvement Act (IDEA), enacted in 1990 and reauthorized in 2004 as P.L.108-446, mandates special education services for youth with special needs. There is a specific reference in this legislation to youth with disabilities being involved in transition planning and also having a written transition plan as part of their Individualized Education Plan (Luecking & Wittenburg, 2009).

IDEA is specific to the education system, and there are other examples of policy within this system that address transition issues through special education legislation. In the United Kingdom, the Special Educational Needs Code of Practice (DfES/581/2001) requires multiagency planning for students with special needs starting at the age of 14. In Canada, many provinces require transition plans for students with special needs, but there is variation. This mandate is at the provincial rather than national level, because education is primarily the responsibility of the provinces. This is an example of how a lack of national policy can act as a barrier to youth with disabilities because the variation in legislation across the country results in inconsistencies in practices.

Legislation specific to other systems and services can also indirectly impact transitions to adulthood for youth with disabilities. For example, in the United States, there is Section 504 of the Rehabilitation Act (amended in 1998 by P.L. 93-516), the Ticket to Work and Work Incentive Improvement Act (P.L. 106-170), and the No Child Left Behind Act of 2001 (P.L. 107-110). Table 1-3 lists similar types of related legislation in other countries.

There is some evidence emerging that legislation is having a positive impact (Luecking & Wittenburg, 2009); however, some studies about the impact of policy on the experiences and outcomes of youth with disabilities report that legislation alone is not enough (Community Living Research Project, 2006). Furthermore, there is a call for policy to address all aspects of transitions to adulthood, and not just one specific area, such as education or health (Committee on Disability in America, 2007; LDAC, 2007). To date, the evidence shows that parents and families of youth with multiple disabilities often have to coordinate several systems on their own, such as education and health care, as the professionals within different systems rarely collaborate (Repetto, Gibson, Lubbers, Gritz, & Reiss, 2008). It is important for occupational therapists to be knowledgeable about legislation related to all systems that can influence adult transitions if they want to provide effective supports to their clients and families.

To conclude this section on environmental factors, it is important to note that it was purposefully organized to discuss environmental supports and barriers together. Although past literature has tended to present environmental factors as either supports or barriers (see Table 1-2), we are learning that any one factor can be perceived as either a barrier or a support. For example, the attitudes and expectations of others (i.e., parents, service providers, and community members) can be a support or a barrier for a youth's development of self-determination. The amount of continuity and consistency between pediatric and adult services can also be supportive if it meets the needs of clients, or a barrier if the services are vastly different. The perception of an environmental factor as a barrier versus support appears to depend on the interaction or fit between personal and environmental factors. If there is a good fit, then a person perceives an environmental factor to be a support, such as collaborative and consistent service delivery. If the fit between person and environment is poor, then there is a perception of a barrier (e.g., low expectations and discriminatory attitudes toward youth with disabilities). This idea about person-environment fit resonates with occupational therapists and is explored in more detail later in this chapter.

Evidence About "Occupation" Components

Within the transition literature, the term *domain* is typically used to refer to the different types of occupations in which young adults are expected to engage. Four primary domains are cited in the literature: employment, education, living arrangements, and socialization/community

Table 1-3.
Useful Links for Occupational Therapists: Government Policy, Legislation, and Reports Related to Transitions to Adulthood for Youth With Disabilities

Broad Legislation About Rights of All Persons With Disabilities	
United States	Americans with Disabilities Act (ADA) (P.L. 110-325), www.ada.gov
Canada	Canadian Charter of Rights and Freedoms
	http://laws-lois.justice.gc.ca/eng/charter
	By province, for example: Accessibility for Ontarians with Disabilities Act (AODA) (2005). www.aoda.ca
United Kingdom	Disability Discrimination Act (DDA) 2005 and Disability Equality Duty (DED) www.legislation.gov.uk/ukpga/2005/13/contents
Australia	National Disability Agreement (NDA)—1/1/09
	www.fahcsia.gov.au/sa/disability/progserv/govtint/Pages/policy-disability_agreement.aspx
	Disability Discrimination Act 1992 www.comlaw.gov.au/Series/C2004A04426
Legislation That Specifically Focuses on Adult Transitions	
United States	Individuals with Disabilities Education Act (IDEA) (Reauthorized 2004)
	http://idea.ed.gov/explore/home
United Kingdom	Autism Act (2009), www.legislation.gov.uk/ukpga/2009/15/contents
Education System Legislation That Includes Transition to Adulthood Issues	
United States	IDEA—*see above*
Canada	By province: for example, in Ontario: The Education Act—Ontario Regulation 464/97—and Education Amendment Act (Bill 82) (1980). www.e-laws.gov.on.ca/html/regs/english/elaws_regs_970464_e.html
United Kingdom	Special Educational Needs Code of Practice (DfES/581/2001) www.education.gov.uk/publications/eOrderingDownload/DfES%200581%20200MIG2228.pdf
Australia	Disability Standards for Education (2005)
	www.deewr.gov.au/Schooling/Programs/Documents/Disability_Standards_for_Education_2005_pdf.pdf
Examples of Legislation Related to Employment and Rehabilitation Systems	
United States	Rehabilitation Act (amended in 1998-P.L. 93-516)
	www2.ed.gov/policy/speced/reg/narrative.html
	Ticket to Work and Work Incentive Improvement Act (P.L. 106-170) www.workworld.org/wwwebhelp/ticket_to_work_and_work_incentives_improvement_act_of_1999.htm
	No Child Left Behind Act (P.L. 107-110) www2.ed.gov/policy/elsec/leg/esea02/index.html
Examples of Legislation Related to Employment and Rehabilitation Systems for Persons With Disabilities	
Canada	Employment Equity Act (1995)
	www.chrc-ccdp.ca/employment_equity/default-eng.aspx
	Vocational Rehabilitation of Disabled Persons Act (1985)
	http://laws.justice.gc.ca/eng/acts/V-3/index.html

activities. These fit well with the domains of occupation that are outlined in the AOTA Practice Framework (Vroman, 2010).

Employment Domain

Within the employment domain, most literature has focused on "school-to-work." Recently the term *school-work transition* has been used to represent a contextual shift in this transition, as young adults are returning to school after working, making the transition a more cyclical process (Thiessen, 2002). The rate of employment for youth with all types of conditions is usually lower than the general average (Altshuler et al., 2008; Billstedt, Gillberg, & Gillberg, 2005; CNIB, 2002; Janus, 2009; LDAC, 2007). The NLTS-2 identified some condition-specific trends related to employment (Wagner et al., 2005). For example, engagement in work was most common for youth with learning disabilities or speech, visual, or other health impairments: more than three-fourths of youth in these categories were engaged. In contrast, youth with intellectual impairments, multiple disabilities, autism, and orthopedic impairments had the lowest rates of work engagement.

Work is a highly valued occupation in most societies. It typically holds meaning for individuals in terms of financial reward, contribution to society, and/or personal identity (Braveman, 2012). Many occupational therapists address employment in some form (paid or volunteer) in their work with clients. Chapters 4 and 6 in this book provide examples of occupational therapy practice in relation to this domain of adult transitions.

Education Domain

The education domain includes both secondary and post-secondary systems. The literature stresses the importance of starting transition planning early in high school when services are free and accessible (Izzo & Lamb, 2003). Youth with psychiatric disorders and learning disabilities often do not complete high school and are therefore at high risk of not meeting adult role expectations (Hollar, 2005; LDAC, 2007; Vander Stoep et al., 2000). Recent articles challenge educators and others to focus more on transition planning and career development rather than just job-finding skills (Cameto et al., 2004). Other reviews identify the importance of post-secondary education for successful adult outcomes (Figure 1-2) and the need for careful transition planning to ensure success (Killean & Hubka, 1999; Wagner et al., 2006). Chapter 5 touches on occupational therapy practice for youth with disabilities in transition to post-secondary education.

Living Arrangements

Living arrangements is a domain that has not been studied in great depth. Leiter and Waugh (2009) found that young adults with disabilities are twice as likely to still be living with parents after the age of 30. The delay in establishing an independent residence was also found in studies of youth with learning, emotional, hearing, visual, physical, and speech impairments (Donkervoort, Wiegerink, Van Meeteren, Stam, & Roebroeck, 2009; Janus, 2009). Leiter and Waugh (2009) identified three key factors that influence living arrangements for all young adults: educational and economic opportunities, changes in norms regarding co-residence with parents, and family resources and supports. They add that the need for care assistance for youth with disabilities can also impact living arrangements. Janus (2009) reported that youth with severe disabilities face the additional challenge of managing personal assistants if they want to live on their own.

> Amanda was diagnosed with schizophrenia at age 17 and had to drop out of high school. For several years, she stayed at home while the professionals tried to find the best medication for her. She also received counseling and cognitive-behavioral treatment during this time. As time passed, she was able to take her remaining high school credits online. She then enrolled in a legal secretary program at college and requested support and accommodation through the disability services office. She had learned how to ask for support when needed and was managing her medications well on her own. She knew that college could be stressful for her, so she decided to continue to live at home with her parents instead of going into residence. Her parents loaned her the money to buy a used car for transportation.

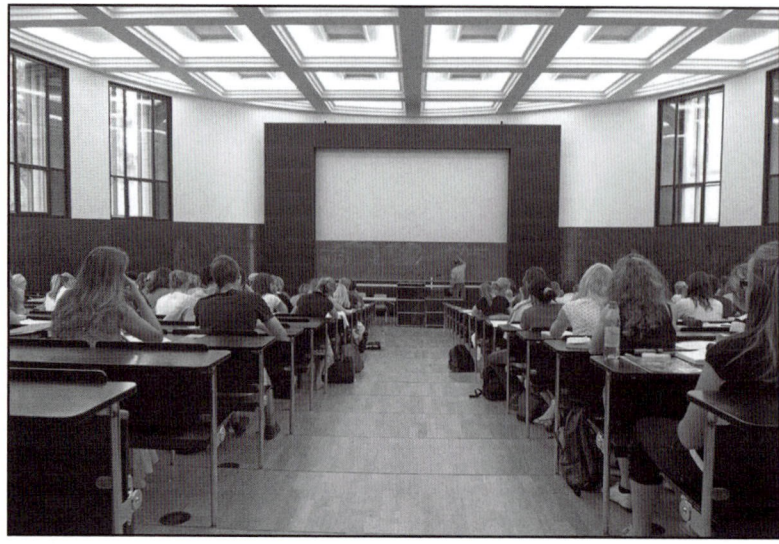

Figure 1-2. Participation in post-secondary education can be an important occupation for young adults.

The literature from several countries supports call for further research in this area and the need to identify a range of options for young people (and their parents) who want to live away from the family home (Blacher, 2001). The concept of *independent living* is explored in relation to occupational therapy practice in Chapter 3.

Social and Community Life Domain

Social and community life domain covers a broad range of transition outcomes and activities, including community recreation and leisure activities (Figure 1-3), social relationships, sexuality, marriage, and parenting. Studies have described poor social outcomes for youth with different types of conditions, such as fewer or poor quality close friendships and few intimate relationships (Clegg, Hollis, Mawhood, & Rutter, 2005; Durkin & Conti-Ramsden, 2007; Janus, 2009; Seltzer et al., 2004; Stewart et al., 2006). Environmental factors can influence an individual's social relationships, as many people have false perceptions and attitudes, such as the belief that people with disabilities are asexual (Janus, 2009). This domain is acknowledged as one that does not receive enough attention (Armstrong et al., 2003; Cooney, 2002). Chapter 7 provides an example of occupational therapy practice in relation to socialization and leisure.

Evidence About Person-Environment-Occupation Interactions and the Complexity of Transitions

Researchers are beginning to focus on interactions and complexities involved in transitions to adulthood. For example, disability was found to interact with other forms of disadvantage, such as ethnicity, poverty, and immigrant status (Burchardt, 2004). Another study found that having a disability and completing secondary education influences future employment outcomes (Vander Stoep et al., 2002). However, knowledge about how these interactions really happen and how they vary among different groups of youth is limited (Burchardt, 2004; Vander Stoep et al., 2002).

Recently, an interactional/multidimensional study about the influence of type and severity of disability on transition outcomes focused on the acquisition of adult social roles. Researchers

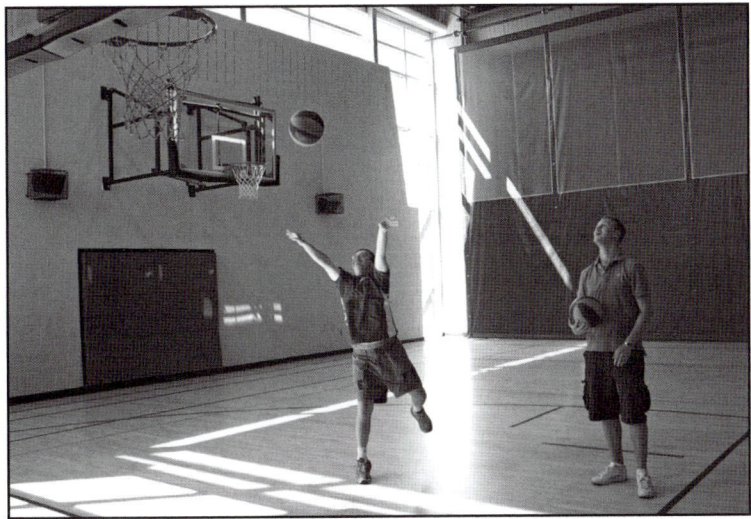

Figure 1-3. A casual game of basketball can provide social opportunities.

found that while severity of a development disability was an important factor, activity limitations and opportunities in the environment were also part of the picture (Van Naarden Braun et al., 2006). These ideas fit well with current occupational therapy views and models of practice.

As mentioned previously, experts have recognized that the label of "barrier" versus "support" often depends on the fit between person and environment—a good fit is perceived as a support or facilitator, and a poor fit is viewed as a barrier or risk factor (Stewart et al., 2008). This concept has received increased attention, as personal and environmental factors have been shown to naturally occur in interaction with each other (Rigby & Letts, 2003). In the past decade, research about transitions to adulthood for youth with disabilities has provided new evidence about the interactive nature of different person and environmental factors, such as the parent-youth relationship (Berzin, 2010). Youth with cognitive or multiple disabilities have been found more likely to have a dependent relationship with their families (Wells et al., 2003). The presence of a severely function-limiting disability can influence a family's ability to invest in the education and employment of their child; thus, the intergenerational transmission of family status can be affected (Wells et al., 2003). In another longitudinal study, the type of impairment and level of care a youth required influenced the parents' level of optimism about the future (Wagner et al., 2005; Wagner et al., 2006).

Interactions between youth with disabilities and others' attitudes have also been studied. In a study about the experiences of males with muscular dystrophy (Gibson, Young, Upshur, & McKeever, 2007), the term *embodied marginalization* (p. 511) was used to describe the interaction between low expectations of youth and the experience of being excluded. Kerka (2002) suggested that underemployment of youth with disabilities was due in part to biased attitudes of others, such as low expectations and overprotectiveness. Views of disability and sexuality were found to be influenced by societal myths that people with disabilities are asexual (Neufeld, Klingbeil, Bryen, Silverman, & Thomas, 2002).

Other person-environment interactions that have been studied recently are related to services and systems. For example, Hanson (2003) found that the expectations of independence in adult services influenced the level of responsibility that parents had to assume for their young adult with disabilities. Within health care services, a lack of professional knowledge and information about the needs of young adults with chronic disabilities was found to influence a person's access to quality health care (Young et al., 2007, 2009).

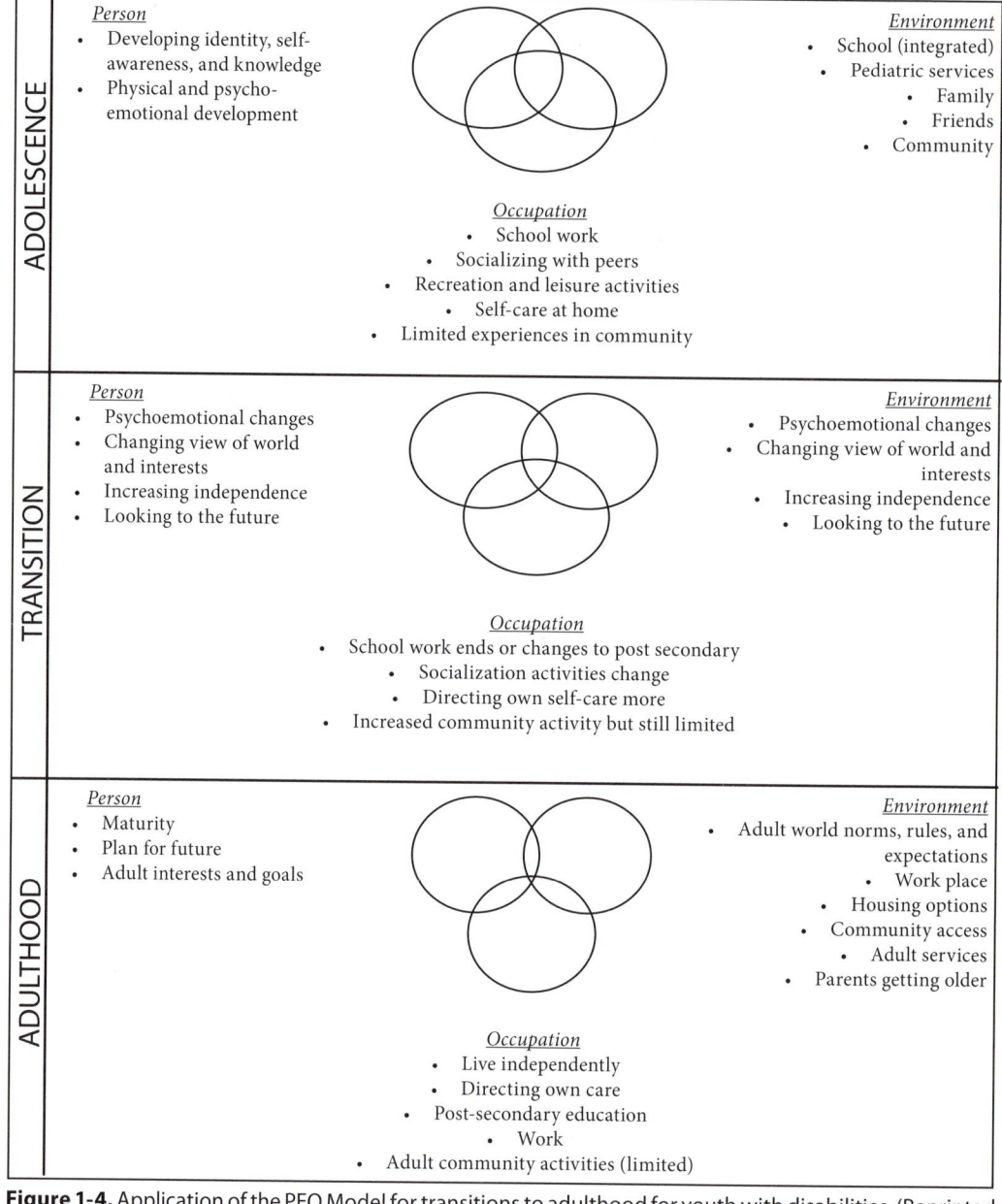

Figure 1-4. Application of the PEO Model for transitions to adulthood for youth with disabilities. (Reprinted with permission from Stewart, D., Law, M., Rosenbaum, P., & Willms, D. [2001]. A qualitative study of the transition to adulthood for youth with disabilities. *Physical and Occupational Therapy in Paediatrics, 21*[4], 3-22.)

Occupational therapists are not likely to find these research findings surprising. We can use our current professional theories and models to explain many of these interactions and complexities. For example, we can use the PEO Model (Law et al., 1996) to demonstrate how the interactions between various factors, as identified in the studies described previously, can result in a positive or negative outcome. Figure 1-4 demonstrates how the PEO Model was used in a qualitative study to depict the transition process of youth with physical disabilities (Stewart et al., 2001). This study found that many adolescents with disabilities and their parents felt that they were "falling off a cliff" (p. 12) when they graduated from high school and were discharged from pediatric services.

The multiple changes in environments and expectations of others in the adult world created a wide gap between PEO. Strategies and supports were needed, including occupational therapy services, to improve the PEO fit. Some of the personal stories in this chapter's boxed asides come from this study, which took place more than 10 years ago—it seems that little has changed since then.

Research about transitions to adulthood for youth with disabilities is entering into a phase of studying the effectiveness of different practice models and supports. Now that we know the factors that influence transition, we can put these together in different ways and find out what combination works best. There is some recent evidence of the effectiveness of specific transition programs for specific populations of youth. For example, Grant and Pan (2011) reviewed five transition programs in Canada for youth with chronic health conditions and found that some (but not all) of these programs have conducted evaluations to demonstrate their effectiveness. In the United States, one program used an evidence-based approach to develop and evaluate a socio-ecological model for transition readiness (Schwartz, Tuchman, Hobbie, & Ginsberg, 2011). Currently, however, there is insufficient evidence to conclude that any one practice model is best for all youth and all systems (Rapley & Davidson, 2010). This finding is not surprising, given the complexity of the transition process.

A critical element for studying the effectiveness of any transition program or service is the identification and measurement of the outcomes of the program. To date, qualitative research has identified a shift in understanding about the outcomes that matter to youth, families, and service providers (Stewart et al., 2008). In the past, outcomes focused more on specific markers of adulthood in the domains of employment, education, living situation, marriage, and becoming a parent. Current studies have identified outcomes of participation, citizenship, relationships, making a contribution to community and society, and quality of life. These types of outcomes fit better with the dreams and aspirations of youth with all types of disability and functional capacities (Stewart et al., 2009). They also fit with current occupational therapy outcomes related to occupational performance and enablement (AOTA, 2008; Townsend & Polatajko, 2007).

Evidence About Occupational Therapy

There is little research evidence about the effectiveness of occupational therapy services and supports for youth with disabilities in transitions to adulthood. Some evaluations of transition programs may include occupational therapy as part of a multidisciplinary transition team.

To date, the literature about occupational therapy specifically has been primarily descriptive, providing information about roles, practice processes, and case scenarios for occupational therapists working in this field. Recent textbooks about pediatric occupational therapy practice include a chapter on transition to adulthood, which acknowledges its importance within practice (Crabtree & Sherwin, 2011; Law & Stewart, 2010; Sample, Bundy, Lane, & Cordier, 2012; Spencer, 2010). The authors who write about occupational therapy roles in this area of practice describe various assessment and intervention strategies within the broad goal of "supporting health and participation in life through engagement in occupation" (AOTA, 2008, p. 626). Occupational therapists often work as related services personnel on a collaborative team within schools providing direct service, education, and consultation to individual clients, groups of youth, and school staff (Law & Stewart, 2010; Spencer, 2010). There are some descriptions of occupational therapy practice in the community with organizations, such as businesses, community agencies, and other professional services (Crabtree & Sherwin, 2011; Spencer, 2010).

Most of the research articles about occupational therapy and transitions to adulthood have used survey methods to study the involvement and perceptions of occupational therapists working in the school system. Three separate surveys have reported low and inconsistent involvement of occupational therapists in transition planning with students in high schools (Kardos & White, 2005; Mankey, 2011; Spencer, Emery, & Schneck, 2003). One of the major barriers to involvement was a lack of awareness about the role of occupational therapy in transition planning. The findings and conclusions from these studies support the call for practitioners to increase their knowledge about the systems in which they work (including education, social services, mental health, and health care) in order to understand and articulate the unique contributions of occupational therapy for transition planning (Gibson et al., 2010; Orentlicher, 2007).

Summary and Critique of Research Evidence

There is relatively strong evidence from different types of studies about personal and environmental factors that influence the transition process, and also about youths' occupational experiences within the domains of employment and education (much less for domains of living arrangements and socialization). There is growing evidence about how these various factors of PEO (domains) interact together. The research evidence is helping to inform service providers about the key elements for best practice—what factors will make a difference, and what is working so far. The current challenges with the research evidence is that it is still silo'd, or segregated, within different systems and for specific youth populations. Recent evidence is pointing us toward more integrated and collaborative research that acknowledges the common processes and outcomes for youth with all types of disabilities in all types of systems.

For occupational therapists, the evidence about multidisciplinary transition programs may be useful, but we do not yet know if our services are making a difference in the lives of youth with disabilities. What can occupational therapists use to guide our practice and decision making? Right now, we need to use the current best available research evidence and augment it with solid theories and models. It is interesting to note that there is no one theory or model that addresses all aspects of transition services and supports—and this is not surprising given the complexities involved. Several theoretical perspectives should be considered by occupational therapists working in this field. Theories and models from three different, yet related, fields appear to be most relevant to occupational therapy practice:

1. Theories and models about development
2. Theories and models about disability
3. Theories and models about occupation

Theories and Models About Development

Current theories on development focus on understanding individuals within their personal, social, cultural, and generational contexts (Lerner, 2002; Lerner & Castellino, 2002). The interactions between person and environment during the developmental process are dynamic in nature and are conceptualized by terms, such as *lifecourse* (Elder, Johnson & Crosnoe, 2003). Recent literature speaks of a transactional developmental process whereby a person is constantly changing, and the changed individual then interacts with his or her human and other environments in a constantly evolving way (Lerner, 2002).

A lifecourse perspective covers the journey through life from start to finish and takes a world view of individuals in an active relationship with their environments (Leiter & Waugh, 2009). A lifecourse approach supports research findings about the transition to adulthood for youth with disabilities, which suggests that the preparation for this transition needs to start much earlier than adolescence. For example, children of elementary school age can begin to work on their self-determination skills by directing other people, such as educational assistants, to help them with tasks that they cannot complete on their own, such as getting dressed. This will enhance their preparation for future adult roles of directing attendants or personal support workers to assist with personal care.

Elaborating on a lifecourse approach, Halfon and Hochstein (2002) combined this approach and theories about health to describe a lifecourse health development model that explains health trajectories over a person's lifetime. This model views health as a dynamic, multifaceted phenomenon that influences a person's functioning. This is a model that is worthy of attention by occupational therapists.

Recently, the term *emerging adulthood* (Arnett, 2004) has been suggested to describe a new stage in the lifecourse of an individual that is typically marked by the end of high school. Many young people in their late teens and early 20s feel they are neither teenagers nor adults. The concept of emerging adulthood has been connected to youth with disabilities, citing additional challenges, such as extended dependency on parents (Jordan & McDonagh, 2007). However, the application of this concept to youth with disabilities requires more study.

There is also a call for an increased focus on positive development throughout adolescence and young adulthood (Hawkins et al., 2011). One study found that positive development is characterized by change and suggests that future research needs to focus on supportive factors that build a youth's capacity for positive functioning during adult transitions (Hawkins et al., 2011).

> Robert has a learning disability, but with appropriate accommodations and supports in high school, he achieved an A average, which enabled him to be accepted into the university program of his choice. He wanted to study kinesiology and ultimately work in the sports medicine field. He found out in the first few months of university that the demands and expectations were very different from high school. He had originally decided not to register with the disability office as he thought he could manage on his own. But he was finding it hard to keep up with the fast pace of the lectures and the large amount of writing involved in the courses. He met with a disability specialist and was told that he would first need a new psychoeducational assessment, as his first assessment was 5 years old. However, the specialist suggested that he speak with his course instructors about his learning disability and ask for informal accommodations until the new assessment was completed and a formal plan for accommodations could be put into place. The specialist also recommended some simple technology that would enable him to record lectures and organize his written work. Robert was pleased to find that all instructors were willing to let him record lectures and gave him extra time on tests and exams, even though he did not have a formal letter from the disability office yet.

Developmental theories and models are being incorporated into new theories about occupational development (Humphry, 2009; Polatajko et al., 2007). Humphry (2009) suggests that occupational therapists can shift our focus from development of the individual to development of occupation. Occupational development takes a contextual perspective to conceptualize changes over time in person and environment. Humphry (2009) proposes that three interlinked change mechanisms take place as a child/youth performs an occupation. These three mechanisms include societal resources, interpersonal influences, and the dynamics of doing the occupation. This builds on interactional theories and models about development, adding in the importance of occupation as a way to connect person and environment. Occupational therapists therefore can contribute to the ongoing conceptual understanding of developmental transitions.

Theories and Models About Disability

Traditionally, there have been two opposing views of disability. Within a medical model, disability has been considered to be a problem within the person, but disability advocates and researchers have provided an alternative view of disability with the social model (Masala & Petretto, 2011). In a social model, disability is viewed as the result of environmental barriers, such as lack of accessibility and discriminatory attitudes (Oliver, 1983). In the past few decades, models

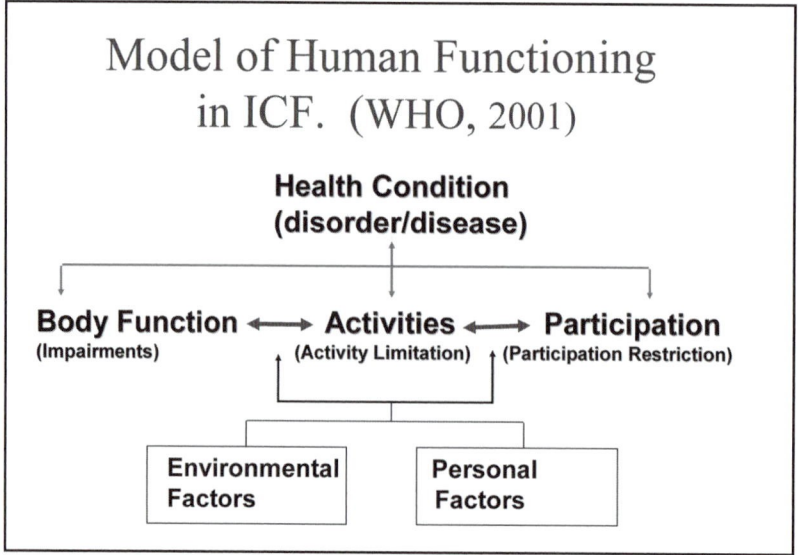

Figure 1-5. The model of human functioning in the ICF (WHO, 2001). (Reprinted with permission from the World Health Organization [WHO]. [2001]. *International classification of functioning, disability and health.* Geneva: Switzerland.)

of disability have presented an interactional view that recognizes the mutual and reciprocal influences of environment and person in dynamic interaction. This view is articulated in the current definition of disability by the World Health Organization (WHO): "…a complex phenomenon, reflecting an interaction between features of a person's body and features of the society in which he or she lives" (2011, p. 1).

The model of human functioning (Figure 1-5) developed by the WHO (2001) as part of the *International Classification of Functioning, Disability and Health* (ICF) (WHO, 2001), emphasizes the relationship between the biopsychosocial elements of a person, including his or her health condition, and contextual factors that influence participation in everyday activities. Other disability theories and models offer an interactional perspective, such as the Disability Creation Process (Fougeyrollas, Cloutier, Bergeron, Côté, & St Michel, 1998) and versions of the Nagi model (Brandt & Pope, 1997). The models can all contribute to clarifying our conceptual understanding of adult transitions.

Priestly (2001) has connected concepts of disability and lifecourse to explore the trajectories of persons with disabilities. Differences in lifecourse trajectories for people with and without disabilities are explained in relation to experiences, expectations, and institutional elements in the environment. This approach fits with the dynamic and interactional frameworks described above and is worthy of further study in relation to adult transitions for youth with disabilities.

Theories and Models About Occupation

Concepts of occupation, occupational performance, and engagement are part of all current theories and models that are the foundation of occupational therapy practice (AOTA, 2008; Polatajko et al., 2007). It is not the intent of this chapter to review all of the current occupational therapy models, but a brief overview of the concepts and theories that are relevant to the transition to adulthood for youth with disabilities can provide some guidance to occupational therapists working in this field.

The concept of occupation is central to our practice (AOTA, 2008; Townsend & Polatajko, 2007). The formal models and theories about occupation identify three major concepts of PEO (Christiansen, Baum & Bass-Haugen, 2005; Dunn, Brown, & McGuigan, 1994; Kielhofner, 2008;

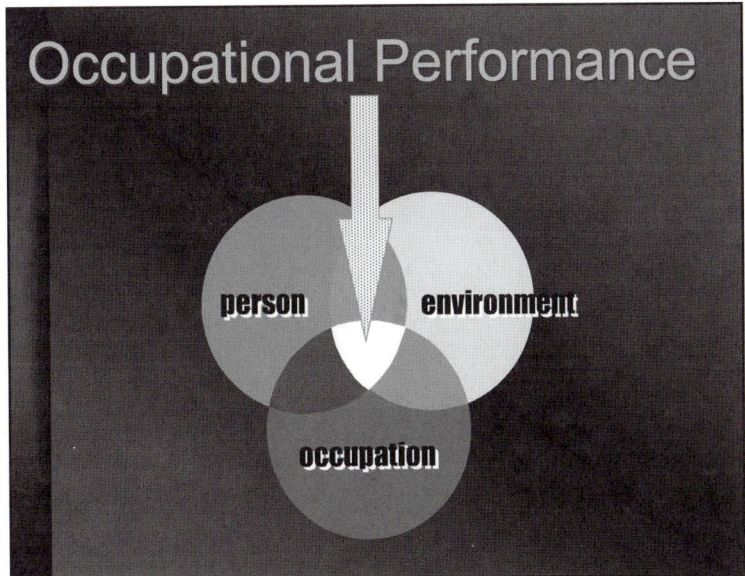

Figure 1-6. PEO Model. (Reprinted with permission from Law, M., Cooper, B., Strong, S., Stewart, D., Rigby, P., & Letts, L. [1996]. The Person-Environment-Occupation Model: A transactive approach to occupational performance. *Canadian Journal of Occupational Therapy, 63*[1], 9-23.)

Law et al., 1996; Schkade & Schultz, 1992; Velde & Fidler, 2002). Different occupational therapy models represent the relationship between these major concepts in different ways, but they all recognize the dynamic nature of the relationships between concepts (Brown, 2009). Terms such as *occupational performance* and *occupational performance and engagement* are often used to describe the result or outcome of a transaction between PEO (AOTA, 2008; Townsend & Polatajko, 2007). In this book, the PEO Model (Law et al., 1996) (Figures 1-6 and 1-7) is used as the primary conceptual framework, but any other occupational therapy model could be substituted to guide the occupational therapist's reasoning and decision making.

Blair (2000) wrote about the centrality of occupation during life transitions, including the transition to adulthood. The author suggests that knowledge from occupational science can be synthesized with theories and research from lifespan developmental psychology to contribute new ideas to the study of life transitions (Blair, 2000). Wright and Sugarman (2009) discuss transitions within a lifecourse perspective and note that a subjective definition of transition, in which a person's self-perception of change is recognized, fits with the client-centered approach of our profession.

Conclusion

The three theoretical perspectives reviewed in this chapter connect concepts about occupational therapy and developmental transitions to adulthood for youth with disabilities. Some common themes are evident from this review:

> ≫ The new theories and models in all three areas are interactive/transactional in nature, recognizing that human experience is based on relationships.

> ≫ All theories and models acknowledge dynamic, changing processes at work in all transitions.

> ≫ All theories and models are taking a more holistic functional view of an individual's life—moving away from components to broad concepts of participation, citizenship, occupation, and lifecourse development.

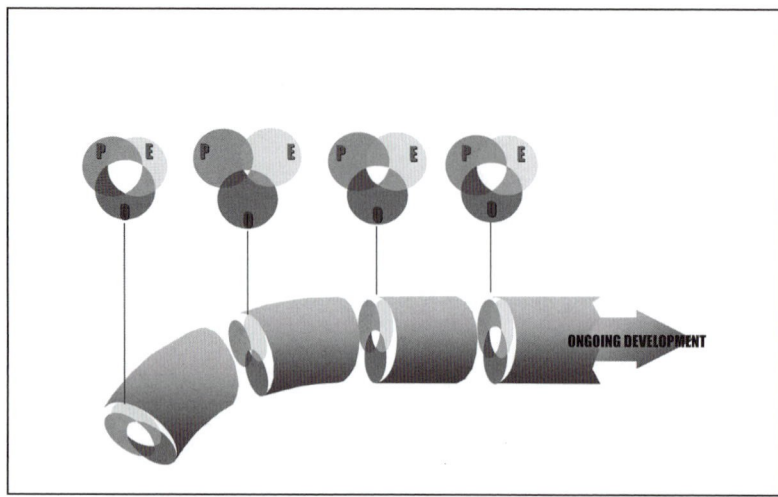

Figure 1-7. PEO model through the lifespan. (Reprinted with permission from (Law, M., Cooper, B., Strong, S., Stewart, D., Rigby, P., & Letts, L. (1996). The Person-Environment-Occupation Model: A transactive approach to occupational performance. *Canadian Journal of Occupational Therapy, 63*(1), 9-23.)

» Individualized, client-centred/person-centered approaches to practice are supported by these theories and models in all three areas.

These common themes demonstrate that there is an excellent fit between occupational therapy models and the theoretical concepts related to transitions to adulthood for youth with disabilities. This theoretical evidence, therefore, supports an active role for occupational therapists on transition teams and in developing services. When these theories are merged with the research evidence reviewed previously, some fundamental principles for occupational therapy practice with youth with disabilities in transition to adulthood emerge:

» Provide occupation-based assessment and intervention strategies to ensure that all services and supports are holistic, strengths-based, developmentally appropriate, and client/person-centered.

» Explore interactions/transactions of PEO rather than each component separately.

» Think beyond individual clients to populations and organizations that can influence, or be influenced by, the transition process. Work collaboratively with team and community members, and always include youth and parents in program planning.

» Start addressing transition issues with clients early—in childhood and through adolescence—using a lifecourse approach. Ask clients and his or her parents regularly about his or her vision and dreams for the future.

Five chapters in this book demonstrate how these principles are put into action for different occupations and settings and with different populations of youth. But first there is one more important issue to address if we want occupational therapists to have the skills and resources to be recognized as essential members of transition teams and programs. Occupational therapists must be able to synthesize their theoretical knowledge in a way that can be understood by others. We need to be able to interpret and explain relevant theories and models in our practice to provide solid rationale for the unique contribution that we can make and the unique perspective that we bring to clients, families, team members, administrators, and funders. And this is not always easy for occupational therapists. The McMaster Lens for Occupational Therapists (Salvatori, 2006) is presented in the next chapter as a resource that guides us to connect our theoretical concepts with practice. "The Lens," as it is commonly called, in Chapter 2 provides a framework for our clinical reasoning which enables us to explain and demonstrate our unique perspective in the field of transition to adulthood. It can also guide our planning and decision making as we build evidence about the effectiveness of our work with youth with disabilities.

Review Questions

1. Summarize and compare traditional and current views about transitions to adulthood. How does the occupational therapy view relate to them?

2. Define and describe self-determination and its role/influence on transition outcomes.

3. What are the different "domains" of occupation?

4. What models and theories can occupational therapists use to guide his or her practice and decision making?

5. What are some of the fundamental principles in occupational therapy practice for youth with disabilities in the transition to adulthood?

References

Algozzine, B., Browder, D., Karvonen, M., Test, D. W, & Wood, W. M. (2001). Effects of interventions to promote self-determination for individuals with disabilities. *Review of Educational Research, 71*(2), 219-277.

Alpern, C. S., & Zager, D. (2007). Addressing communication needs of young adults with autism in a college-based inclusion program. *Education and Training in Developmental Disabilities, 42*(4), 428-436.

Altshuler, S. J., Mackelprang, R. W., & Baker, R. L. (2008). Youth with disabilities: A standardized self-portrait of how they are faring. *Journal of Social Work in Disability & Rehabilitation, 7*(1), 1-18.

American Occupational Therapy Association (AOTA) (2008). *Occupational therapy practice framework: Domain and process* (2nd ed.). Bethesda, MD: American Occupational Therapy Associaton Press.

Armstrong, K. H., Dedrick, R. F., & Greenbaum, P. E. (2003). Factors associated with community adjustment of young adults with serious emotional disturbance: A longitudinal analysis. *Journal of Emotional and Behavioral Disorders, 11*(2), 66-76.

Arnett, J. J. (2004). *Emerging adulthood: The winding road from the late teens through the twenties.* New York, NY: Oxford University Press.

Baltodano, H. M., Mathur, S. R., & Rutherford, R. B. (2005). Transition of incarcerated youth with disabilities across systems and into adulthood. *Exceptionality, 13*(2), 103-124.

Bartlett, D. J., Hanna, S. E., Avery, L., Stevenson, R. D., & Galuppi, B. (2010). Correlates of decline in gross motor capacity in adolescents with cerebral palsy in gross motor function classification system levels III to V: An exploratory study. *Developmental Medicine & Child Neurology, 52*(7), 155-160. doi:10.1111/j.1469-8749.2010.03632.x

Beresford, B. (2004). On the road to nowhere? Young disabled people and transition. *Child: Care, Health, and Development, 30*(6), 581-587.

Berge, J. M., Patterson, J. M., Goetz, D., & Milla, C. (2007). Gender differences in young adults' perceptions of living with cystic fibrosis during the transition to adulthood: A qualitative investigation. *Families, Systems, and Health, 25*(2), 190-203.

Berzin, S. C. (2010). Vulnerability in the transition to adulthood: Defining risk based on youth profiles. *Children and Youth Services Review, 32*(4), 487-495.

Billstedt, E., Gillberg, I. C., & Gillberg, C. (2005). Autism after adolescence: Population-based 13- to 22-year follow-up study of 120 individuals with autism diagnosed in childhood. *Journal of Autism and Developmental Disorders, 35*(3), 351-360.

Binks, J. A., Barden, W. S., Burke, T. A., & Young, N. L. (2007). What do we really know about the transition to adult-centered health care? A focus on cerebral palsy and spina bifida. *Archives of Physical Medicine and Rehabilitation, 88*(8), 1064-1073.

Blacher, J. (2001). Transition to adulthood: Mental retardation, families, and culture. *American Journal on Mental Retardation, 106*(2), 173-188.

Blackorby, J., & Wagner, M. (1996). Longitudinal post-school outcomes of youth with disabilities: Findings from the national longitudinal study. *Exceptional Children, 62*(5), 339-413.

Blackstock, C., Bruyere, D., & Moreau, E. (2006). *Many hands, one dream: Principles for a new perspective on the health of First nations, Inuit and Métis children, and youth.* Ottawa, Ontario, Canada: Canadian Pediatric Society. Retrieved April 16, 2011 from www.manyhandsonedream.ca/english/manyhands-principles.pdf

Blair, S. E. E. (2000). The centrality of occupation during life transitions. *British Journal of Occupational Therapy, 63*(7), 231-239.

Blue-Banning, M., Turnbull, A. P., & Pereira, L. (2002). Hispanic youth/young adults with disabilities: Parents' visions for the future. *Research and Practice for Persons with Severe Disabilities, 27*(3), 204-219.

Bowe, F. G. (2003). Transition for deaf and hard-of-hearing students: A blueprint for change. *Journal of Deaf Studies and Deaf Education, 8*(4), 485-493.

Brandt, E. N., & Pope A. M. (Eds.). (1997). *Enabling America: Assessing the role of rehabilitation science and engineering.* Washington, DC: National Academy Press.

Braveman, B. (2012). Work in the modern world. The history and current trends in workers, the workplace and working. In B. Braveman & J. J. Page (Eds.), *Work: Promoting participation and productivity through occupational therapy* (pp. 2-27). Philadelphia, PA: F. A. Davis.

Brown, C. E. (2009). Ecological models in occupational therapy, In E. B. Crepeau, E.S. Cohn, & B.A. Boyt Schell (Eds.), *Willard and Spackmans' occupational therapy* (11th ed.), New York, NY: Lippincott Williams & Wilkins.

Burchardt, T. (2004). Aiming high: The educational and occupational aspirations and of young disabled people. *Support for Learning, 19*(4), 181-186.

Cameto, R., Levine, P., & Wagner, M. (2004). *Transition planning for students with disabilities: A special topic report of findings from the national longitudinal transition study-2 (NLTS2).* Washington, DC: National Center for Special Education Research.

Canadian National Institute for the Blind (CNIB) (2002). *The status of Canadian youth who are blind or visually impaired: A study of lifestyles, quality of life, and employment.* Toronto, Ontario, Canada: Canadian National Institute for the Blind.

Carter, E. W., Trainor, A., Owens, L., Sweden, B., & Sun, Y. (2010). Self-determination prospects of youth with high-incidence disabilities: Divergent perspectives and related factors. *Journal of Emotional and Behavioral Disorders, 18*(2), 67-81.

Caton, S., & Kagan, C. (2007). Comparing transition expectations of young people with moderate learning disabilities with other vulnerable youth and with their non-disabled counterparts. *Disability and Society, 22*(5), 473-488.

Chambers, C. R., Hughes, C., & Carter, E. W. (2004). Parent and sibling perspectives on the transition to adulthood. Education and Training in Developmental Disabilities, 39(2), 79-94.

Christiansen, C., Baum, D., & Bass-Haugen, J. (Eds.). (2005). *Occupational therapy: Performance, participation, and well-being* (3rd ed.). Thorofare, NJ: SLACK Incorporated.

Clegg, J., Hollis, C., Mawhood, L., & Rutter, M. (2005). Developmental language disorders—a follow-up in later adult life. Cognitive, language, and psychosocial outcomes. *Journal of Child Psychology and Psychiatry, 46*(2), 128-149. doi:10.1111/j.1469-7610.2004.00342.x

Colver, A., Dickinson, H., & SPARCLE Group. (2010). Study protocol: Determinants of participation and quality of life of adolescents with cerebral palsy: A longitudinal study (SPARCLE2). *BMC Public Health, 10*(1), 280.

Committee on Disability in America. (2007). Health care transitions for young people. In M. J. Field, & A. M. Jette (Eds.), *Future of disability in America* (pp. 4-1). Washington, DC: The National Academies Press.

Community Living Research Project. (2006). *Young adults with developmental disabilities: Transition for high school to adult life. Literature and initial program review.* Vancouver, BC: School of Social Work and Family Studies, University of British Columbia.

Cooney, B. F. (2002). Exploring perspectives on transition of youth with disabilities: Voices of young adults, parents, and professionals. *Mental Retardation, 40*(6), 425-435.

Crabtree, L., & Sherwin, A. B. (2011). Begin with the end in mind: Promoting mental health, social participation, and self-determination in the transition from school to adult life. In S. Bazyk (Ed.), *Mental health promotion, prevention, and intervention with children and youth: A guiding framework for occupational therapy.* Bethesda, MD: American Occupational Therapy Association Press.

Darrah, J., Magill-Evans, J., & Galambos, N. L. (2010). Community services for young adults with motor disabilities—a paradox. *Disability and Rehabilitation, 32*(3), 223-229.

Davis, M., & Sondheimer, D. L. (2005). State child mental health efforts to support youth in transition to adulthood. *The Journal of Behavioral Health Services and Research, 32*(1), 27-42.

Donkervoort, M., Wiegerink, D. J., Van Meeteren, J., Stam, H. J., & Roebroeck, M. E. (2009). Transition to adulthood: Validation of the Rotterdam transition profile for young adults with cerebral palsy and normal intelligence. *Developmental Medicine and Child Neurology, 51*(1), 53-62.

Dunn, W., Brown, C., & McGuigan, A. (1994). The ecology of human performance: A framework for considering the impact of context. *American Journal of Occupational Therapy, 48*(7), 595-607.

Durkin, K., & Conti-Ramsden, G. (2007). Language, social behavior, and the quality of friendships in adolescents with and without a history of specific language impairment. *Child Development, 78*(5), 1441-1457. doi:10.1111/j.1467-8624.2007.01076.x

Elder, G. H., Johnson, M. K., & Crosnoe, R. (2003). The emergence and development of life course theory. In J.T. Mortimer & M.J. Shanahan (Eds.). *Handbook of the Life Course.* New York, NY: Kleuwer.

Field, S., & Hoffman, A. (2002). Preparing youth to exercise self-determination. *Journal of Disability Policy Studies, 13*(2), 114-119.10.1177/10442073020130020701

Foster, S., & MacLeod, J. (2004). The role of mentoring relationships in the career development of successful deaf persons. *Journal of Deaf Studies and Deaf Education, 9*(4), 442-458.

Fougeyrollas, P., Cloutier, R., Bergeron, H., Côté, J., &. St Michel, G. (1998). *The Quebec Classification Disability Creation Process, Québec, International Network on Disability Creation Process (INDCP)/CSICIDH*. Retrieved August 31, 2011 from www.ripph.qc.ca/?rub2=2&rub=6&lang=en.

Frank, A. R., & Sitlington, P. L. (2000). Young adults with mental disabilities—Does transition planning make a difference? *Education and Training on Mental Retardation and Developmental Disabilities, 35*(2), 119-134.

Gibson, B. E., Young, N. L., Upshur, R. E. G., & McKeever, P. (2007). Men on the margin: A bourdieusian examination of living into adulthood with muscular dystrophy. *Social Science and Medicine, 65*(3), 505-517. doi: 10.1016/j.socscimed.2007.03.043

Gibson, R. W., Nochajski, S. M., Schefkind, S., Myers, C., Sage, J., & Marshall, A. (2010). The role of occupational therapy in transitions throughout the lifespan. *Occupational Therapy Practice, 15*(11), 11-14.

Gorter, J. W., Stewart, D., & Woodbury-Smith, M. (2011). Youth in transition: Care, health and development. *Child: Care, Health, and Development, 37*(6), 757-763.

Goupil, G., Tassé, M. J., Garcin, N., & Doré, C. (2002). Parent and teacher perceptions of individualised transition planning. *British Journal of Special Education, 29*(3), 127-135.

Grant, C., & Pan, J. (2011). A comparison of five transition programs for youth with chronic illness in Canada. *Child: Care, Health and Development, 37*(6), 815-820.

Grove, B., & Giraud-Saunders, A. (2003). Connecting with connexions: The role of the personal adviser with young people with special educational and support needs. *Support for Learning, 18*(1), 12-17.

Halfon, N., & Hochstein, M. (2002). Life course health development: An integrated framework for developing health, policy, and research. *Milbank Quarterly, 80*(3), 433-479. doi:10.1111/1468-0009.00019

Hamdani, Y., Jetha, A., & Norman, C. (2011). Systems thinking perspectives applied to healthcare transition for youth with disabilities: A paradigm shift for practice, policy, and research. *Child: Care, Health, and Development, 37*(6), 806-814. doi: 10.1111/j.1365-2214.2011.01313.x

Hanson, M. J. (2003). Twenty-five years after early intervention: A follow-up of children with Down syndrome and their families. *Infants and Young Children, 16*(4), 354-365.

Hawkins, M. T., Letcher, P., Sanson, A., O'Connor, M., Toumbourou, J. W., & Olsson, C. (2011). Stability and change in positive development during young adulthood. *Journal of Youth and Adolescence, 40*(11), 1436-1452.

Hetherington, S. A., Durant-Jones, L., Johnson, K., Nolan, K., Smith, E., Taylor-Brown, S., & Tuttle, J. (2010). The lived experiences of adolescents with disabilities and their parents in transition planning. *Focus on Autism and Other Developmental Disabilities, 25*(3), 163-172.

Hitchings, W. E., Luzzo, D. A., Ristow, R., Horvath, M., Retish, P., & Tanners, A. (2001). The career development needs of college students with learning disabilities: In their own words. *Learning Disabilities: Research and Practice, 16*(1), 8-17.

Hollar, D. (2005). Risk behaviors for varying categories of disability in NELS: 88. *Journal of School Health, 75*(9), 350-358. doi:10.1111/j.1746-1561.2005.tb06695.x

Horsman, M., Suto, M., Dudgeon, B., & Harris, S. R. (2010). Growing older with cerebral palsy: Insiders' perspectives. *Pediatric Physical Therapy, 22*(3), 296-303. doi:10.1097/PEP.0b013e3181eabc0f

Humphry, R. (2009). Occupation and development: A contextual perspective. In E. B. Crepeau, E. S. Cohn, & B. A. Boyt Schell (Eds.), *Willard and Spackman's occupational therapy* (11th ed., pp. 22-32). New York, NY: Lippincott Williams & Wilkins.

Izzo, M. V., & Lamb, P. (2003). Developing self-determination through career development activities: Implications for vocational rehabilitation counselors. *Journal of Vocational Rehabilitation, 19*(2), 71-78.

Janus, A. L. (2009). Disability and the transition to adulthood. *Social Forces, 88*(1), 99-120.

Jivanjee, P., Kurzich, J. M., & Gordon, L. J. (2009). The age of uncertainty: Parent perspectives on the transitions of young people with mental health difficulties into adulthood. *Journal of Child and Family Studies, 18*(4), 435-446.

Jonikas, J. A., Laris, A., & Cook, J. A. (2003). The passage to adulthood: Psychiatric rehabilitation service and transition-related needs of young adult women with emotional and psychiatric disorders. *Psychiatric Rehabilitation Journal, 27*(2), 114-121.

Jordan, A., & McDonagh, J. E. (2007). Recognition of emerging adulthood in UK rheumatology: The case for young adult rheumatology service developments. *Rheumatology, 46*(2),188-191.

Kardos, M., & White, B. P. (2005). The role of the school-based occupational therapist in secondary education transition planning: A pilot survey study. *American Journal of Occupational Therapy, 59*(2), 173-180.

Kerka, S. (2002). *Learning disabilities and career development*. Practice application brief no. 20. Retrieved February 20, 2011 from http://www.ericacve.org/pubs.asp

Kielhofner, G. (2008). *Model of human occupation: Theory and application* (4th ed.). Philadelphia, PA: Lippincott, Williams & Wilkins.

Killean, E., & Hubka, D. (1999). *Working towards a coordinated national approach to services, accommodations and policies for post-secondary students with disabilities: Ensuring access to higher education and career training*. Ottawa, Ontario, Canada: National Educational Association of Disabled Students (NEADS).

King, G. A., Brown, E. F., & Smith, L. K. (2003). *Resilience: Learning from people with disabilities and the turning points in their lives*. Westport, CT: Praeger.

King, G., Cathers, T., Miller Polgar, J., MacKinnon, E., & Havens, L. (2000). Success in life for older adolescents with cerebral palsy. *Qualitative Health Research, 10*(6), 734-749.

Kirby, A., Sugden, D., Beveridge, S., & Edwards, L. (2008). Developmental co-ordination disorder (DCD) in adolescents and adults in further and higher education. *Journal of Research in Special Educational Needs, 8*(3), 120-131. doi:10.1111/j.1471-3802.2008.00111.x

Kraus de Camargo, O. (2011). Systems of care: Transition from the bio-psycho-social perspective of the International Classification of Functioning, Disability and Health. *Child: Care, Health and Development, 37*(6), 792-900.

Law, M., Cooper, B., Strong, S., Stewart, D., Rigby, P., & Letts, L. (1996). The Person-Environment-Occupation Model: A transactive approach to occupational performance. *Canadian Journal of Occupational Therapy, 63*(1), 9-23.

Law, M., & Stewart, D., (2010). Transitions to adulthood. In K. J. Dodd, C. Imms, & N. F. Taylor (Eds.), *Physiotherapy and occupational therapy for people with cerebral palsy* (pp. 230-244). London, England: MacKeith Press.

Learning Disabilities Association of Canada (LDAC). (2007). *Putting a Canadian face on learning disabilities* (PACFOLD). Ottawa, Ontario, Canada: Learning Disabilities Association of Canada.

Lehman, C. M., Clark, H. B., Bullis, M., Rinkin, J., & Castellanos, L. A. (2002). Transition from school to adult life: Empowering youth through community ownership and accountability. *Journal of Child and Family Studies, 11*(1), 127-141.

Leiter, V., & Waugh, A. (2009). Moving out: Residential independence among young adults with disabilities and the role of families. *Marriage and Family Review, 45*(5), 519-537.

Lerner, R. M. (2002). *Concepts and theories of human development.* Mahwah, NJ: Lawrence Erlbaum Associates.

Lerner, R. M., & Castellino, D. R. (2002). Contemporary developmental theory and adolescence: Developmental systems and applied developmental science. *Journal of Adolescent Health, 31*(6), 122-135.

Luecking, R. G. & Wittenburg, D. (2009). Providing supports to youth with disabilities transitioning to adulthood: Case descriptions from the Youth Transition Demonstration. *Journal of Vocational Rehabilitation, 30*(3), 241-251.

Levine, P., & Nourse, S. W. (1998). What follow-up studies say about post-school life for young men and women with learning disabilities: A critical look at the literature. *Journal of Learning Disabilities, 31*(3), 212-233.

Lounds, J., Seltzer, M. M., Greenberg, J. S., & Shattuck, P. T. (2007). Transition and change in adolescents and young adults with autism: Longitudinal effects on maternal well-being. *American Journal of Mental Retardation, 112*(6), 401-417. doi: 0895-8017-112-6-401 [pii] 10.1352/0895-8017(2007)112[401:TACIAA]2.0.CO;2

Magill-Evans, J., Wiart, L., Darrah, J., & Kratochvil, M. (2005). Beginning the transition to adulthood: The experiences of six families with youths with cerebral palsy. *Physical and Occupational Therapy in Pediatrics, 25*(3), 19-36.

Mankey, T. (2011). Occupational therapists' beliefs and involvement with secondary transition planning. *Physical and Occupational Therapy in Pediatrics, 31*(4), 345-358.

Martorell, A., Gutierrez-Recacha, P., Pereda, A., & Ayuso-Mateos, J. L. (2008). Identification of personal factors that determine work outcome for adults with intellectual disability. *Journal of Intellectual Disability Research, 52*(12), 1091-1101.

Masala C, & Petretto, D. R. (2011). Models of disability. In: J. H. Stone & M. Blouin (Eds.), *International Encyclopedia of Rehabilitation.* Available online: http://cirrie.buffalo.edu/encyclopedia/en/article/135/

McConachie, H. (2011). Improving mental health transitions for young people with autism spectrum disorder. *Child: Care, Health and Development, 37*(6), 764-766.

McGuire, J., & McDonnell, J. (2008). Relationships between recreation and levels of self-determination for adolescents and young adults with disabilities. *Career Development for Exceptional Individuals, 31*(3), 154-163.

Mull, C. A., & Sitlington, P. L. (2003). The role of technology in the transition to post-secondary education of students with learning disabilities: A review of the literature. *Journal of Special Education, 37*(1), 26-33.

Neufeld, J. A., Klingbeil, F., Bryen, D. N., Silverman, B., & Thomas, A. (2002). Adolescent sexuality and disability. *Physical Medicine and Rehabilitation Clinicc of North America, 13*(4), 857-873.

Oliver, M. (1983). *The politics of disability paper given at the the annual general meeting of the disability alliance.* Retrieved from www.leeds.ac.uk/disability-studies/archiveuk

Orentlicher, M. L. (2007). Transition from school to adult life. In L. L. Jackson (Ed.), *Occupational therapy services for children and youth under IDEA* (3rd ed., pp. 187-211). Bethesda, MD: American Occupational Therapy Association Press.

Polatajko, H. J., Davis, J., Stewart, D., Cantin, N., Amoroso, B., Purdie, L., & Zimmerman, D. (2007). Specifying the domain of concern: Occupation as core. In E. A. Townsend & H. J. Polatajko (Eds.), *Enabling occupation II: Advancing an occupational therapy vision for health, well-being & justice through occupation* (pp. 13-86). Ottawa, Ontario, Canada: CAOT Publications ACE.

Powers, K., Geenen, S., & Powers, L. E. (2009). Similarities and differences in the transition expectations of youth and parents. *Career Development for Exceptional Individuals, 32*(3), 132-144.

Powers, K., Hogansen, J., Geenan, S., Powers, L. E., & Gil-Kashiwabara, E. (2008). Gender matters in transition to adulthood: A survey study of adolescents with disabilities and their families. *Psychology in the Schools, 45*(4), 349-364.

Powers, L. E. (2001). *Take charge for the future.* Portland, OR: Center on Self-Determination, Oregon Health Sciences University.

Priestly, M. (Ed.). (2001). *Disability and the life course: Global perspectives*. Cambridge, UK: Cambridge University Press.

Rapley, P., & Davidson, P. M. (2010). Enough of the problem: A review of time for health care transition solutions for young adults with a chronic illness. *Journal of Clinical Nursing, 19*(3-4), 313-323.

Reinehr, T., Dobe, M., Winkel, K., Schaefer, A., & Hoffmann, D. (2010). Obesity in disabled children and adolescents: An overlooked group of patients. *Deutsches Arzteblatt International, 107*(15), 268-275. doi:10.3238/arztebl.2010.0268.

Reiss, J. G., Gibson, R. W., & Walker, L. R. (2005). Health care transition: Youth, family, and provider perspectives. *Pediatrics, 115*(1), 112-120.

Repetto, J. B., Gibson, R. W., Lubbers, J., Gritz, S., & Reiss, J. (2008). A statewide study of knowledge and attitudes regarding health care transition. *Career Development for Exceptional Individuals, 31*(1), 5-13.

Rigby, P., & Letts, L. (2003). Environment and occupational performance: Theoretical considerations. In L. Letts, P. Rigby, & D. Stewart (Eds.), *Using environments to enable occupational performance*. Thorofare, NJ: SLACK Incorporated.

Saigal, S., Stoskopf, B., Streiner, D., Boyle, M., Pinelli, J., Paneth, N., & Goddeeris, J. (2006). Transition of extremely low-birth-weight infants from adolescence to young adulthood: Comparison with normal birth-weight controls. *The Journal of the American Medical Association, 295*(6), 667-675.

Salvatori, P., Jung B., Missiuna C., Stewart D., Law, M., & Wilkins, S. (2006). *The McMaster lens for occupational therapists*. Hamilton, Ontario, Canada: McMaster University.

Sample, P. L., Bundy, A. C., Lane, S. J., & Cordier, R. (2012). Transitioning to adulthood. What will I be when I grow up? In S. L. Lane & A. C. Bundy (Eds.), *Kids can be kids: A childhood occupations approach* (pp. 102-124). Philadelphia, PA: F. A. Davis.

Schkade, J. K., & Schultz, S. (1992). Occupational adaptation: Toward a holistic approach to contemporary practice, part 1. *American Journal of Occupational Therapy, 46*(9), 829-837.

Schwartz, L. A., Tuckman, L. K., Hobbie, W. L., & Ginsberg, J. P. (2011). A social-ecological model of readiness for transition to adult-oriented care for adolescents and young adults with chronic health conditions. *Child: Care, Health, and Development, 37*(6), 883-895.

Seltzer, M. M., Shattuck, P., Abbeduto, L., & Greenberg, J. S. (2004). Trajectory of development in adolescents and adults with autism. *Mental Retardation and Developmental Disabilities Research Review, 10*(4), 234-247. doi:10.1002/mrdd.20038

Shikako-Thomas, K., Majnemer, A., Law, M., & Lach, L. (2008). Determinants of participation in leisure activities in children and youth with cerebral palsy: Systematic review. *Physical and Occupational Therapy in Pediatrics, 28*(2), 155-169. doi:10.1080/01942630802031834

Spencer, J. E., Emery, L. J., & Schneck, C. M. (2003). Occupational therapy in transitioning adolescents to post-secondary activities. *American Journal of Occupational Therapy, 57*(4), 435-443.

Spencer, K. C. (2010). Transition services: From school to adult life. In J. Case-Smith & J. C. O'Brien (Eds.), *Occupational therapy for children* (6th ed.). St. Louis, MO: Elsevier.

Stewart, D. (2003). Peer mentorship as an environmental support for adolescents and young adults with disabilities. In L. Letts, P. Rigby, & D. Stewart (Eds.), *Using environments to enable occupational performance*. Thorofare, NJ: SLACK Incorporated.

Stewart, D., Freeman, M., Law, M., Healy, H., Burke-Gaffney, J., Forhan, M.,...Guenther, S. (2009). *The best journey to adult life for youth with disabilities: An evidence-based model and best practice guidelines for the transition to adulthood for youth with disabilities*. Hamilton, Ontario, Canada: McMaster University.

Stewart, D., Law, M., Rosenbaum, P., & Willms, D. (2001). A qualitative study of the transition to adulthood for youth with disabilities. *Physical and Occupational Therapy in Pediatrics, 21*(4), 3-22.

Stewart, D., Law, M., Young, N., Healy, H., Forhan, M., Burke-Gaffney, J., & Freeman, M. (2008). *Understanding the transitional tensions of youth with disabilities in Canada: Identifying key research gaps*. Penultimate Report to Human Resources Social Development Canada (HRSDC). Hamilton, Ontario, Canada: McMaster University. Unpublished document.

Stewart, D., Stavness, C., King, G., Antle, B., & Law, M. (2006). A critical appraisal of literature reviews about the transition to adulthood for youth with disabilities. *Physical and Occupational Therapy in Pediatrics, 26*(4), 5-24.

Thiessen, V. (2002). *Policy research issues for Canadian youth: School-work transitions*. Ottawa, Ontario, Canada: Applied Research Branch, Strategic Policy, Human Resources Development Canada.

Townsend, E. A., & Polatajko, H. J. (Eds.), (2007). *Enabling occupation II: Advancing an occupational therapy vision for health, well-being, and justice through occupation*. Ottawa, Ontario, Canada: CAOT Publications ACE.

Turnbull, A. P., & Turnbull, R. (2006). Self-determination: Is a rose by any other name still a rose? *Research and Practice for Persons with Severe Disabilities (RPSD), 31*(1), 83-88.

Vander Stoep, A., Weiss, N. S., McKnight, B., Beresford, S. A., & Cohen, P. (2002). Which measure of adolescent psychiatric disorder—diagnosis, number of symptoms, or adaptive functioning—best predicts adverse young adult outcomes? *Journal of Epidemiology and Community Health, 56*(1), 56-65.

Van Naarden Braun, K., Yeargin-Allsopp, M., & Lollar, D. (2006). A multi-dimensional approach to the transition of children with developmental disabilities into young adulthood: The acquisition of adult social roles. *Disability and Rehabilitation, 28*(15), 915-928.

Velde, B., & Fidler, G. (2002). *Lifestyle performance. A model for engaging the power of occupation.* Thorofare, NJ: SLACK Incorporated.

Vroman, K. (2010). In transition to adulthood: The occupations and performance skills of adolescents. In J. Case-Smith & J. C. O'Brien (Eds.), *Occupational therapy for children* (6th ed.). St. Louis, MO: Elsevier.

Wagner, M., Newman, L., Cameto, R., & Levine, P. (June, 2005). *National Longitudinal Transition Study 2: Changes over time in the early postschool outcomes of youth with disabilities.* Menlo Park, CA: SRI International.

Wagner, M., Newman, L., Cameto, R., Levine, P., & Garza, N. (2006). *An overview of findings from wave 2 of the National Longitudinal Transition Study-2 (NLTS2).* Menlo Park, CA: National Center for Special Education Research.

Wehmeyer, M. L. (2005). Self-determination and individuals with severe disabilities: Reexamining meanings and interpretations. *Research and Practice in Severe Disabilities, 30,* 113-120.

Wehmeyer, M. L., Abery, B., Mithaug, D. E., & Stancliffe, R. (2003). *Theory in self-determination. Foundations for educational practice.* Springfield, IL: Charles C. Thomas Publishing.

Wehmeyer, M., & Palmer, S. B. (2003). Adult outcomes for students with cognitive disabilities three years after high school: The impact of self-determination. *Education and Training in Developmental Disabilities, 38*(2), 131-144.

Wells, T., Sandefur, G. D., & Hogan, D. P. (2003). What happens after the high school years among young persons with disabilities? *Social Forces, 82*(2), 803-832.

Williams-Diehm, K., Wehmeyer, M. L., Palmer, S. B., Soukup, J. H., & Garner, N. W. (2008). Self-determination and student involvement in transition planning: A multivariate analysis. *Journal on Developmental Disabilities, 14*(1), 27-39.

Wright, R., & Sugarman, L. (2009). *Occupational therapy and life course development. A workbook for professional practice.* West Sussex, UK: John Wiley & Sons.

Wright, M., Tancredi, A., Yundt, B., & Larin, H. (2006). Sleep issues in children with physical disabilities and their families. *Physical and Occupational Therapy in Pediatrics, 26*(3), 55-72. doi:10.1080/J006v26n03_05

Wong, M. E. (2004). Higher education or vocational training? some contributing factors to post-school choices of visually impaired students in britain. Part 1, Great Britain. *British Journal of Visual Impairment, 22*(1), 37.

World Health Organization (WHO). (2001). *International classification of functioning, disability and health.* Geneva: Switzerland.

World Health Organization (WHO). (2011). *Disability.* Retrieved October 25, 2011 from http://www.who.int/topics/disabilities/en/

Young, N. L., Barden, W. S., Mills, W. A., Burke, T. A., Law, M., & Boydell, K. (2009). Transition to adult-oriented health care: Perspectives of youth and adults with complex physical disabilities. *Physical and Occupational Therapy in Pediatrics, 29*(4), 345-361.

Young, N. L., Gilbert, T. K., McCormick, A., Ayling-Campos, A., Boydell, K., Law, M.,...Williams, J. I. (2007). Youth and young adults with cerebral palsy: Their use of physician and hospital services. *Archives of Physical Medicine and Rehabilitation, 88*(6), 696-702.

2

The McMaster Lens for Occupational Therapists
Linking Theory to Practice

Mary Law, PhD, FCAOT, FCAHS

Since the 1980s, many new theoretical concepts, frameworks, and practice models have emerged in the occupational therapy literature (American Occupational Therapy Association [AOTA], 2008; Canadian Association of Occupational Therapists [CAOT], 1997; Dunn, Brown, & McGuigan, 1994; Fidler, 1996; Kielhofner, 2008; Law et al., 1996; Townsend & Polatajko, 2007). While there are differences amongst these frameworks and models, they all share a focus on occupation and the ways in which factors within the person and the environment support or hinder participation in occupation. Kathleen Reed has distinguished between two predominant types of models in occupational therapy (Reed & Sanderson, 1999). The first type is the conceptual model, which explains theoretical concepts underlying occupation and occupational therapy. Conceptual models tend to be more generic in focus and do not address specific areas of occupational therapy practice. They are often labeled as *occupation-based models*. The second type is the practice model, which, in contrast, explains how occupational therapy is implemented and often provides guidelines for specific types of evaluation and intervention. They are most often labeled as *frames of reference*.

As theoretical concepts have developed, conceptual and practice models have used concepts and terminology inconsistently. Models often contain concepts and therapy processes that overlap. Because of these challenges, student occupational therapists have difficulty integrating conceptual and practice models into a clear understanding of how theory can be used to guide clinical practice. Similarly, practicing occupational therapists often face this dilemma.

Over the past decade, faculty at McMaster University, who teach theoretical concepts in the occupational therapy master's program, have reviewed the curriculum and focused on effective methods to address the learning needs of our students in this area. In the occupational therapy program, theory about occupation and occupational therapy is introduced in the first semester and knowledge is built through all semesters until graduation. The ultimate goal is to ensure that by the time of graduation, students can use theory to guide practice. In reflecting on how to

Stewart, D. (Ed.)
Transitions to Adulthood for Youth With Disabilities Through an Occupational Therapy Lens (pp. 27-46).
© 2013 SLACK Incorporated

achieve this goal, faculty identified the need to clearly articulate the unique theoretical perspec- tive of occupational therapists. These discussions ultimately led to the development of a guide linking theory to the practice of occupational therapy called the McMaster Lens for Occupational Therapists (Salvatori et al., 2006).

The McMaster Lens for Occupational Therapists is a tool for student occupational therapists and practitioners to guide their thinking about using theory and practice. The Lens represents a metaphor for bringing theory and practice into focus. As a tool for "thinking" (versus "doing"), the Lens does not replace existing occupational therapy conceptual or practice models. Rather, the Lens provides a practical strategy for incorporating existing knowledge and models into everyday practice. In each component of the Lens, examples from existing theoretical literature are used to illustrate their use within the process of occupational therapy practice.

In this book, the McMaster Lens for Occupational Therapists provides an organizational tool for understanding and thinking about transitions to adulthood for youth with disabilities. The component parts of the Lens are described in detail in this chapter along with an example to illus- trate its application. For each component, specific practice questions are provided to guide your thinking about theory and practice. In subsequent chapters, the framework of the Lens is used to organize the information presented, and to demonstrate how it can be used in different situations to guide occupational therapists' thinking and decision making.

Lenses in a Telescope—A Metaphor for Occupational Therapy Practice

Merriam-Webster's Online Dictionary (2005) defines a lens as something that "facilitates and influences perception, comprehension, or evaluation," and also suggests that lenses can be "combined in an optical instrument for forming an image," The McMaster Lens for Occupational Therapists (Figure 2-1) uses multiple lenses brought together as a telescope to represent a meta- phor to describe the process of occupational therapy practice. The telescope consists of a series of eight lenses (occupation, spirituality, development, person-environment-occupation [PEO], theo- retical approach, assessment, treatment, and outcome) that are used by an occupational therapist with each client, whether an individual, a group, or an organization. The fundamental concept in using a telescope as a metaphor is that each lens in the telescope is movable and is adjusted by the occupational therapist to bring the client's unique situation into focus. Such adjustments represent the clinical reasoning and decision making of an occupational therapist throughout the therapeutic process.

Occupational therapy supports a client and family-centered approach to therapy practice (Sumsion & Law, 2006; Townsend & Polatajko, 2007). A fundamental principle of this approach is the focus on the specific needs of each client, group, or organization. Occupational therapists recognize that each client brings specific strengths and needs to a therapy encounter. For example, two youth may have the same diagnosis and functional abilities, but have different patterns of par- ticipation in occupation and live in different environments. The therapeutic approach must build in flexibility to address the unique aspect of each client while also being guided by evidence-based theoretical knowledge.

Each step in the occupational therapy process, such as choosing a theoretical approach, select- ing assessment strategies, and planning a treatment program, requires specific strategies for each client. Guided by conceptual and practice models, the occupational therapist views every client situation through the same series of lenses. However, the lenses are adjusted differently in every situation to reflect the client's unique circumstances and to bring theory and practice into focus. The final image is different for each client but reflects the unique theoretical perspective of occupational therapy. The McMaster Lens for Occupational Therapists represents this unique perspective.

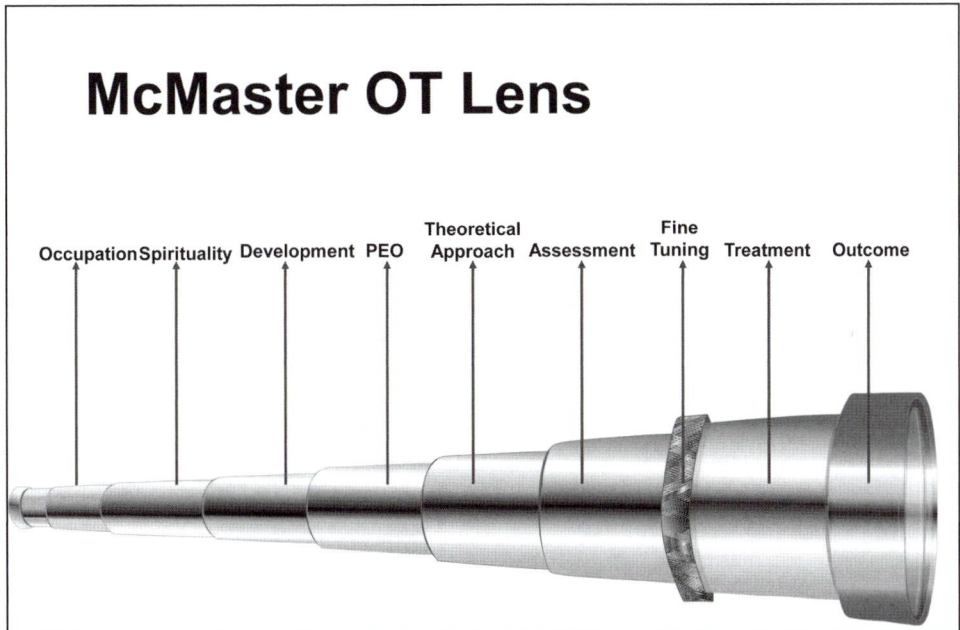

Figure 2-1. The McMaster Occupational Therapy Lens. (Reprinted with permission from Salvatori, P., Jung, B., Missiuna, C., Stewart, D., Law, M., & Wilkins, S. [2006]. *The McMaster lens for occupational therapists.* Hamilton, Ontario, Canada: McMaster University.)

The McMaster Lens for Occupational Therapists is a telescope with eight lenses as well as an adjustment ring for fine tuning. Each lens represents one component of the process by which occupational therapists use theory to guide practice. In every practice encounter, an occupational therapist can use the Lens to guide the therapy process.

The development of the Lens was guided by important theoretical knowledge that has developed within occupational therapy over the past two decades. First, knowledge about clinical reasoning in occupational therapy underlies each component of the Lens. As detailed in work by Mattingly and Fleming (1994), occupational therapists use procedural/scientific, narrative/interactive, ethical, and conditional reasoning to support their decision making during occupational therapy assessment and treatment. These processes of clinical reasoning underpinned the thinking and decision making of therapists during each component of the Lens.

A second important influence on the development of the Lens was the generic model of occupation put forward by McColl and colleagues (2003). As depicted in Figure 2-2, this model puts forward an organizational structure for theories about occupation and occupational performance. The first level consists of the three predominant categories of occupation: self-care, productivity, and leisure. At this level, conceptual theories about occupation help occupational therapists understand the nature and experiences of occupation. Occupation and occupational performance can be facilitated or hindered by factors within the person or the environment. Thus, the other areas of the model described components within the person, and types of environmental factors that have substantial influences on the ways in which daily occupations are carried out. Specific details about the theories within this organizational structure will be discussed in the section on Lens #5.

The Canadian Model of Occupational Performance (CMOP) (CAOT, 1997; Townsend & Polatajko, 2007) influenced the development of specific concepts included in the Lens. In the Canadian Model, spirituality is conceived as "the essence of the self" (CAOT, 1997, p. 42). Spirituality is expressed through each person's unique nature and can be viewed as the way in

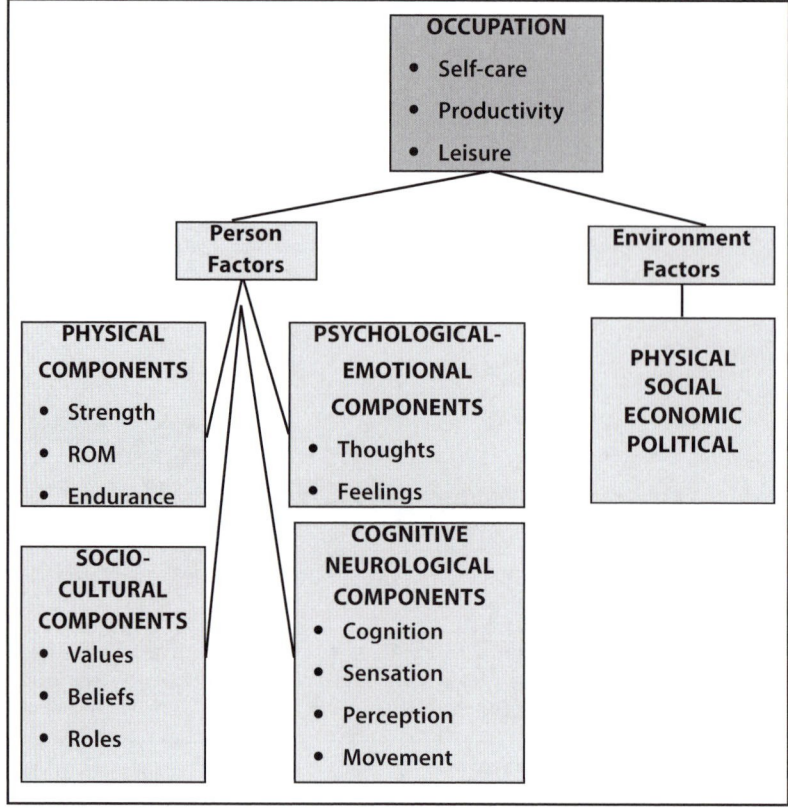

Figure 2-2. The basis for occupational therapy theory: a generic model of occupation. (Reprinted with permission from McColl, M. A., Law, M., Stewart, D., Doubt, L., Pollock, N., & Krupa, T. [2003]. *Theoretical basis of occupational therapy* [2nd ed.]. Thorofare, NJ: SLACK Incorporated.)

which persons find meaning through occupation. As articulated within the CMOP, spirituality may be expressed through religion but is also expressed through a person's experiences, values, and innate qualities. Although controversial, the concept of spirituality is now considered by many occupational therapists around the world as one of the essential ways in which engagement in occupation can be explained.

The unique contribution of occupational therapy is the discipline's focus on the relationship between PEOs in which they carry out these occupations. In the development of the Lens, we have used the PEO Model (Law et al., 1996) to reflect this ecological approach that is central to occupational therapy theory and practice. The PEO concepts are used in the fourth component of the Lens to describe the process of occupational analysis that is a part of every occupational therapy encounter.

Finally, the development of the Lens reflected occupational therapy's focus on client-centered practice. A client may include individuals, groups, agencies, governments, corporations, or others (CAOT, 1997). Client-centered occupational therapy recognizes that clients bring experience and knowledge about their occupations and their needs to each occupational therapy encounter. The principles of client-centred practice are implemented when occupational therapists show "respect for clients, involve clients in decision making, advocate with and for clients in meeting clients' needs, and otherwise recognize clients' experience and knowledge" (CAOT, 1997, p. 49). The therapeutic relationship between the client, his or her family, and the occupational therapist is a collaborative partnership whose goal is to enhance participation in the occupations of everyday life (Law, 1998).

Let us now look at each component of the Lens. For each component, a description of the essential concepts and characteristics of the component are provided. A figure of the pictorial representation of each lens accompanies the description. Questions to guide the reasoning of the occupational therapist for each component of the lens are listed. Finally, the application of the component of the lens to the practice scenario is described.

Lens #1—Practice Scenario

Within this book, each chapter is focused on a specific domain of transition to adulthood for youth with different types of disability and includes individual and group practice scenarios. Therefore, in this chapter, we take a population perspective to the application of the Lens so that readers can explore an example of how the Lens applies to populations of youth. This practice scenario focuses on issues of youth with lifelong disabilities in transition to adulthood within a specific community. Community A is a small city with a population of 90,000 people. Approximately 15% of the population (13,500) in Community A is youth from 12 to 21 years of age. In North America, it is estimated that between 5% to 10% of children and youth have a disability that affects their ability to carry out daily activities (Janus, 2009; Wood, Reiss, Ferris, Edwards, & Merrick, 2010). Thus, there are about 600 to 700 youth with disabilities in Community A. The city council and local recreation, culture, and sport organizations have come together to improve access to outside-of-school activities for all youth. As part of this process, they are examining access for youth with disabilities. They believe that youth who develop healthy participation patterns when they are younger will carry these patterns into adulthood. Together, they have engaged the services of an occupational therapist to assist with this process. We will use this practice scenario to examine how the occupational therapists can work with the city council and local organizations to improve access.

Lens #1—Occupation

The importance of meaningful occupation in the lives of individuals, groups, and organizations is the central tenet of occupational therapy (AOTA, 2008). Occupational therapy conceptual and practice models consistently focus on the importance of occupation and its influence on health and well-being (Townsend & Polatajko, 2007; Watson & Wilson, 2003). Over the past 20 years, the discipline of occupational science has developed to build knowledge about occupation, the experiences of humans as they participate in daily occupations. Without occupation, occupational therapy would not exist. Therefore, occupation is the first and most important lens through which the occupational therapist views the client.

As depicted in Figure 2-3, occupation provides meaning in the lives of every human. Occupation has been defined as "groups of activities and tasks of everyday life, named, organized, and given value and meaning by individuals and culture. Occupation is everything people do to occupy themselves, including looking after themselves (self-care), enjoying life (leisure), and contributing to the social and economic fabric of their communities (productivity)" (CAOT, 1997, p. 34). Other definitions of occupation include "goal-directed pursuits that typically extend over time, have meaning to the performance, and involve multiple tasks," (Christiansen, Baum, & Bass-Haugen, 2005, p. D48) and "daily activities that reflect cultural values, provide structure to living, and meaning to individuals; these activities meet human needs for self-care, enjoyment, and participation in society" (Crepeau, Cohn, & Boyt Schell, 2003, p. 1031).

Occupational therapists around the world have developed descriptive categories to help organize their thinking about occupation. For example, the AOTA, in its Practice Framework, categorizes occupation as "activities of daily living, instrumental activities of daily living, rest and sleep, education, work, play, leisure, and social participation" (AOTA, 2008 p. 630).

In the CMOP (CAOT, 1997), three categories of occupation are described: self-care, productivity, and leisure. Self-care encompasses occupations predominantly focused on the individual that support daily functioning in the areas of activities of daily living and community living. Examples

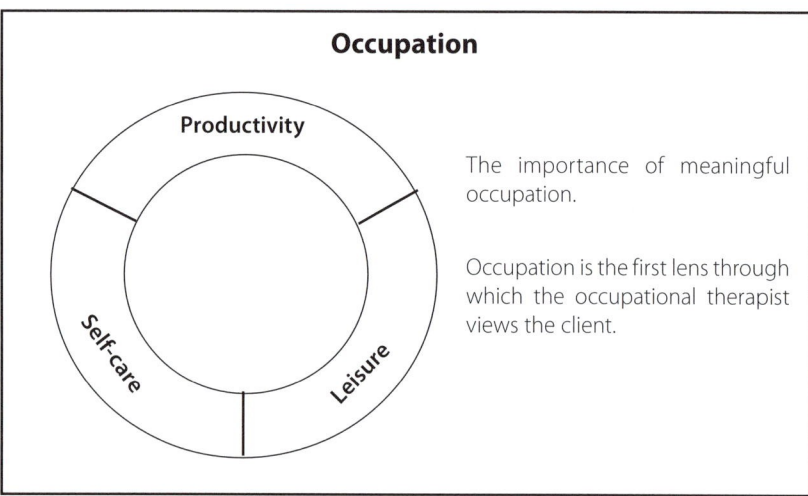

Figure 2-3. The Occupation Lens. (Reprinted with permission from Salvatori, P., Jung, B., Missiuna, C., Stewart, D., Law, M., & Wilkins, S. (2006). *The McMaster lens for occupational therapists.* Hamilton, Ontario, Canada: McMaster University.)

of self-care include personal care, such as eating, bathing, and dressing; household and community occupations, such as shopping, banking, making meals, and gardening; and household and community mobility. Productivity occupations make a "social or economic contribution or provide for economic sustenance" (CAOT, 1997, p. 37). Examples of productivity include education, volunteering, paid work, parenting, and for children, the occupation of play. Such occupations represent our contributions to home, family, community, workplace, or society (McColl et al., 2003, p. 2). Finally, leisure occupations are not obligatory and are participated in for enjoyment (CAOT, 1997). Examples of leisure occupations include socializing with friends, hobbies, physical activities and sports, games, and getting together with family. Participation in leisure occupations is largely influenced by the youth's preferences (King et al., 2006) and includes occupations that may be sedentary or active, social or solitary, creative or technical (McColl et al., 2003, p. 2).

In Figure 2-3, the occupation categories from the Canadian Model are illustrated as an example. These categories could be easily replaced by those from the AOTA Practice Framework or other occupational therapy theoretical models. The most important idea to remember as an occupational therapist working with youth in transition is to begin the occupational therapy process with a focus on occupation. Consideration of the full scope of occupations in which youth participate will enable a holistic approach to occupational therapy treatment.

For the lens of occupation, there are two important questions to be considered by the occupational therapist. Let's consider each question in turn.

1.   What occupation(s) does this client engage in as part of his or her typical daily routine?

Every youth involved in occupational therapy enters this process with a daily repertoire of occupations. Their participation in occupations—which ones, how often, where, and with whom—is the central and first focus of the occupational therapist. Information about the daily routine can be gathered through narrative interview or through an assessment of participation. The specific approach to gathering this information is determined by each occupational therapist after considering the individual(s), the reason for referral, and the practice approach. Through a narrative interview with the client(s), therapists gain information about their experiences with occupation and their daily routine. Standardized assessments can also be used to describe patterns of occupations and participation in occupations. While the purpose of this book is not to detail specific assessments, examples of assessments of participation in occupations for youth include the following standardized measures:

» Canadian Occupational Performance Measure (COPM) (Law et al., 2005): A responsive, individualized outcome measure through which occupational performance issues are identified and measurement of change after therapy intervention is assessed.

» Goal Attainment Scaling (GAS) (Kiresuk, Smith, & Cardillo, 1994): A standardized process through which specific goals are identified and levels of potential achievement within each goal are specified.

» Assessment of Life Habits (LIFE-H) (Noreau, Fougeyrollas & Vincent, 2002): Measures an individual's life habits (regular activities) and social roles within different environments. There are adapted forms for children between the ages of 5 and 13 years (LIFE-H for Children) (Fougeyrollas, Noreau, & Lepage, 2003; Noreau, Lepage, & Boissiere, 2007).

» Children's Assessment of Participation and Enjoyment (CAPE) (King et al., 2004): A questionnaire designed to examine how children and youth between the ages of 6 and 21 years participate in everyday activities outside of their school classes.

» Occupational Performance History Interview II (OPHI-II) Version 2.1, 2004 (Kielhofner et al., 2004; Kielhofner, Mallinson, Forsyth, & Lai, 2001): A historical interview that uses narrative to explore a person's life history, the impact of disability, and the direction in which the person would like to take his or her life.

» School Function Assessment (SFA) (Coster, Deeney, Haltiwanger, & Haley, 1998): A measure of a student's ability to perform functional activities that support or enable participation in an educational program within elementary schools.

2. Which occupation(s) is/are currently difficult for this client to perform?

While knowledge about a youth's daily occupations provides excellent background for understanding issues, the occupational therapist needs to gather specific information about current difficulties with occupations. This step is the most important activity of the occupation component of the Lens. The goal of therapy is to enable persons to engage in the occupations "…that they want to do, need to do, or are expected to do in daily life" (Law et al., 2005, p. 13). Thus, the identification of the occupations with which the young person is experiencing challenges will form the basis for every other component of the Lens.

Lens #2—Practice Scenario

For occupation, there are many different occupations and roles that are typically meaningful and important during the transition to adulthood. Key transition occupations can be organized under the three categories of self-care, productivity, and leisure. For example, self-care occupations can include self-management of personal care activities, medication and health care, life skills, instrumental activities of daily living (IADL), and future community living skills such as transportation, banking, shopping, and housing. Productive occupations can include occupations related to current and future education, voluntary activity, and employment. Leisure occupations can include recreation, socialization, and the development of peer relationships, intimate and sexual relationships, and changing family relationships. Research indicates that the occupations and roles that are important and meaningful to youth with lifelong disabilities are exactly the same for all youth (Stewart et al., 2008).

Within our population-based practice scenario, the occupations that will be of most interest to the youth population in Community A and relate to the specific purpose of the project primarily fit within leisure occupations. In considering access, the occupational therapist ensures that the city council and organizations consider leisure occupations from the broadest perspective, including recreation, culture, and sport occupations. As well, access to volunteer opportunities within the city should be considered.

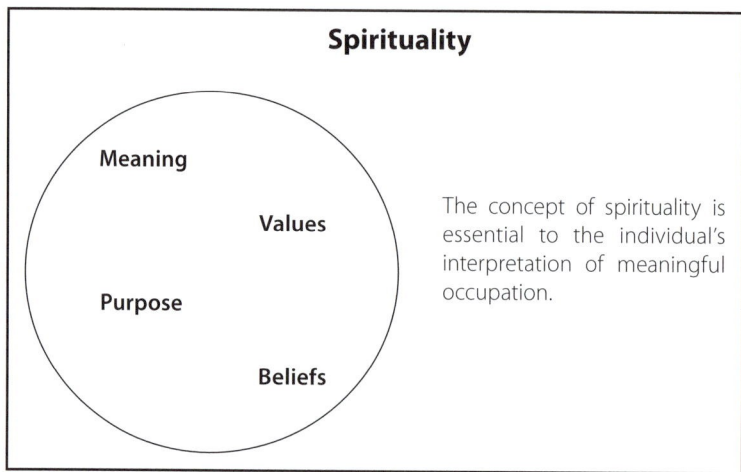

Figure 2-4. The Spirituality Lens. (Reprinted with permission from Salvatori, P., Jung, B., Missiuna, C., Stewart, D., Law, M., & Wilkins, S. [2006]. *The McMaster Lens for Occupational Therapists.* Hamilton, Ontario, Canada.)

Lens #2—Spirituality

The concept of spirituality was included in the Lens (Figure 2-4) because it is considered to be essential to the individual's interpretation of meaningful occupation (CAOT, 1997). Spirituality, within this context, is defined as a source of self-determination and personal control (CAOT, 1997). Within occupational therapy, a secular understanding of spirituality is the most common: spirituality is considered to be "humanistic, rational/empirical, individualistic, and not-corporate/non-institutional" (McColl, 2011, p. 57). One of the main features that appear in most definitions of spirituality is a relationship with meaning or purpose in life, and this feature is one that occupational therapists can relate to most (McColl, 2003).

In recognizing a person's spirituality, occupational therapists provide respect for a person's experiences with occupation and his or her beliefs, values, and goals. Spirituality is shaped by the environment in which persons live, work, and play; their relationships with family, friends, and others; and their religious affiliations if present. The person's sense of spirituality provides meaning to the occupations in which he or she participates every day (CAOT, 1997).

For the lens of spirituality, there is one important question to be considered by the occupational therapist.

1.   What is the meaning/importance/value of these occupations for this client?

Consider the cultural context and groups that this individual belongs to in exploring spirituality (e.g., values of the family, ethnic background, religious affiliations, employment, and/or professional relationships and associations).

Lens #3—Practice Scenario

In considering spirituality, the occupational therapist thinks about the meaning of adult transitions for society, for families, and for youth with lifelong disabilities. In North American communities, transition typically focuses on growing up into responsibility, participating in new occupations, making contributions to society, and managing one's daily life. Transition to adulthood has changed over the years and there is now a more extended period of transition time, from the adolescent years, well into the 20s.

The occupational therapist knows that the period of transition is often challenging for families since it typically includes letting go. During transition, most parents begin to plan for a future without children living in their home. Although youth often return to the family home for periods

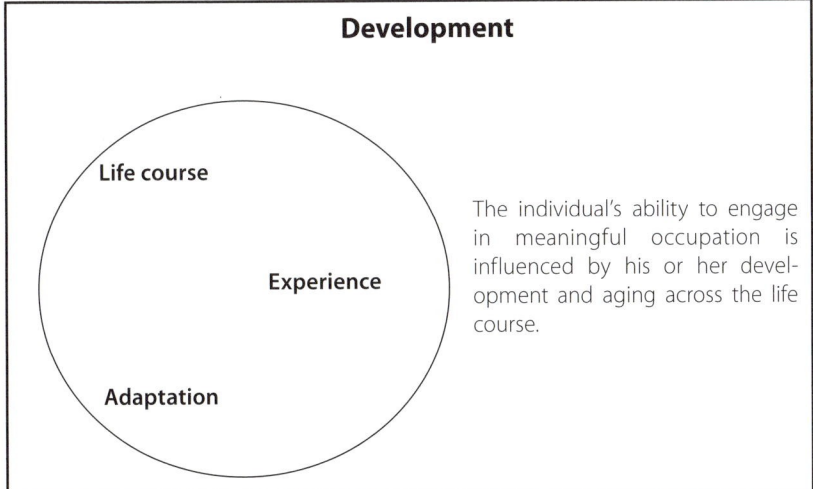

Figure 2-5. The Development Lens. (Reprinted with permission from Salvatori, P., Jung, B., Missiuna, C., Stewart, D., Law, M., & Wilkins, S. [2006]. *The McMaster Lens for Occupational Therapists.* Hamilton, Ontario, Canada: McMaster University.)

of time, most parents expect to be on their own as their adult children move out and have their own lives.

In working with the city and organizations, the occupational therapist will share knowledge about the occupations in which youth with lifelong disabilities typically participate. An essential part of this knowledge is that youth with lifelong disabilities usually value and want to participate in the same occupations as youth without disabilities. The vast majority of youth with lifelong disabilities want to contribute to society, participate in their community, have a job, be in relationship, and move away from his or her parents. However, he or she faces significant barriers in achieving these goals.

Lens #3—Development

A youth's engagement in meaningful occupation is influenced by his or her development. For example, the occupations in which a 13-year-old youth engages are often very different from an 18-year-old who is about to enter college. Development influences engagement in occupations through both biological maturation ("nature") and environmental experience/adaptation ("nurture"). Adolescence is a time of major developmental change. From a dynamic systems perspective, adolescence represents a continuous, ever-changing process of development (Case-Smith, Law, Missiuna, Pollock, & Stewart, 2010).

Occupational therapists working with youth use a developmental perspective to examine the dynamic, evolving interaction between the youth, his or her environment, and chosen occupations. During adolescence, youth will be developing new occupations and leaving behind many of the occupations that they experienced as children.

For the lens of development (Figure 2-5), there are two important and interrelated questions to be considered by the occupational therapist.

1. From a lifecourse perspective, at what stage of development is this client?

Consider both the client's chronological age and current level of functioning, as well as the expectations of this client with regard to the demands of the occupation(s).

2. What are the expectations for this developmental stage?

Consider the cultural and/or societal expectations for the occupation of interest. For example, it is a typical developmental expectation within North American culture for youth in late adolescence to have the capacity to get around in their community independently, either by driving (have a driver's license) or by public transportation.

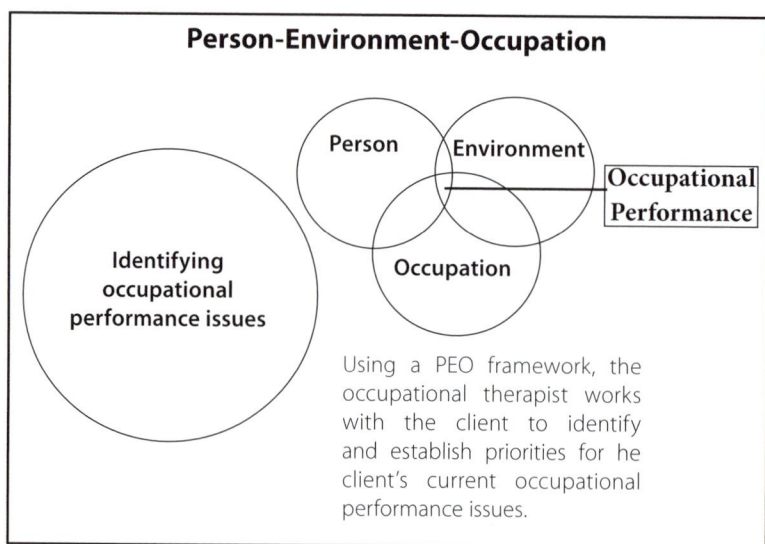

Figure 2-6. The Person-Environment-Occupation Lens. (Reprinted with permission from Salvatori, P., Jung, B., Missiuna, C., Stewart, D., Law, M., & Wilkins, S. [2006]. *The McMaster Lens for Occupational Therapists*. Hamilton, Ontario, Canada: McMaster University.)

Consideration of the fit between the client's developmental level of functioning and the typical developmental expectations of occupations will assist the occupational therapist in addressing relevant and important developmental issues related to the occupational performance of youth with disabilities.

Lens #4—Practice Scenario

From a developmental perspective, we have already discussed the fact that the majority of youth with disabilities want to participate in age-appropriate occupations. The occupational therapist understands and provides information to the city and organizations about typical development and developmental milestones during adolescence and young adulthood. He or she can also provide knowledge about the impact that difficulties in achieving all developmental milestones can have on participation in leisure occupations.

Lens #4—Person-Environment-Occupation

Currently, the hallmark of occupational therapy, regardless of the theoretical approaches used, includes a focus on persons doing occupations within several environments. To emphasize the importance of the continuous relationship between youth, their occupations, and their environments, the fourth component of the Lens centers on this relationship. Within this component of the Lens, the occupational therapist examines the fit/lack of fit between the person's abilities and skills, the demands of the occupation, and the environmental conditions in which the occupation takes place (Law et al., 1996). This process of analyzing these relationships begins from the initial contact and interview with the client.

To illustrate PEO interactions within the Lens, the developers have used the PEO model (Figure 2-6) (Law, 1998; Law et al., 1996). Other overarching occupational therapy conceptual models that include concepts relating PEOs can also be used for this component of the Lens. Examples of other models that can be used for this component include the Canadian Model of Occupational Performance and Engagement (CMOP-E) (Townsend & Polatajko, 2007), the Ecology of Human Performance Model (EHP) (Dunn et al., 1994), and the Model of Human Occupation (MOHO) (Kielhofner, 2008).

The PEO Model focuses on the transactional relationship between PEOs in which these occupations are carried out. In this model, a person is viewed as an integrated whole who incorporates spirituality, social and cultural experiences, and observable occupational performance (Law et al., 1996). Performance components or "client factors" (AOTA, 2008, p. 630) within the person have a significant influence on successful engagement in occupation. The result of the PEO relationship is a person's occupational performance. Occupational performance has both subjective and objective characteristics and reflects the youth's choices of occupations and the way in which to do them.

Occupations are carried out within many different environments. In the PEO Model, environments are defined as those contexts and situations that occur outside individuals and elicit responses from them (Law et al., 1996). Environmental factors that influence occupation include cultural, institutional, physical, and social characteristics of the environment. Environments within the home, work, school, and community provide the context in which occupation takes place.

Occupation has been defined earlier in this chapter. Within the PEO Model, it is important to recognize that occupation places affective, cognitive, and physical demands on the individual performing the occupation. As well, occupations often require that a person use tools or equipment and be able to perform the occupation in different environments. The PEO Model recognizes the complexity of participation in occupation. Occupational therapists use their analytical skills to understand the results of the lack of fit between a person's skills and abilities, the requirements of the occupation, and/or the demands of the environment.

For the Lens component of PEO, the following question is important for the occupational therapist to consider.

1. What are the underlying PEO factors that influence the client's ability to perform these occupations?

Consider how each occupation is typically performed in this client's environment when attempting to explain the client's current occupational performance issues.

Lens #5—Practice Scenario

Using the PEO perspective, the occupational therapist can provide knowledge to the city and organizations about the dynamic, ever-changing nature of transition in leisure occupations. This dynamic nature of occupational performance is illustrated in Figure 2-6. The occupational therapist is an expert in understanding the most significant components of PEO during the transition process. We have already discussed the components of occupation earlier in this chapter. From a person perspective, identity development during late adolescence and early adulthood is a critical personal component. As youth mature and take on more responsibility for their daily occupations, there is the need to learn and develop personal factors that are important in this process. As a youth develops, he or she experiences changes in physical, cognitive, and emotional/affective skills and abilities.

From an environment perspective, the occupational therapist will focus on specific community environments in which recreation, culture, and sport occupations take place. At this stage in the process, the occupational therapist can begin to explore potential environmental barriers and supports that impact the participation of youth in community leisure occupations. Factors within the environment can be both supports and barriers, and this can change rapidly. For example, parents and family can be viewed as a barrier one day, as they are not letting go, and as a support the next day when they provide transportation to a social event.

Lens #5—Theoretical Approach

By the time the occupational therapist reaches Lens #5 in his or her reasoning process, he or she will have: (1) information about the occupations of greatest meaning and concern to the youth and his or her family, (2) considered the developmental stage, and (3) begun the process of thinking about which factors within the PEO are influencing occupational performance. By this point, the

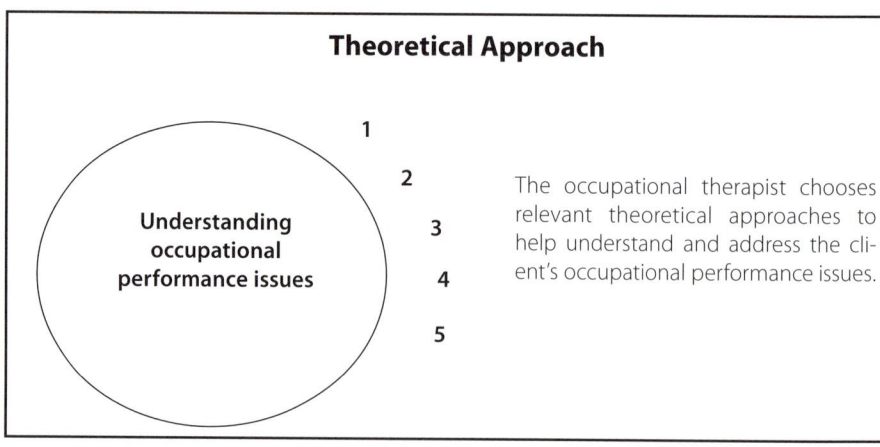

Figure 2-7. The Theoretical Approach Lens. (Reprinted with permission from Salvatori, P., Jung, B., Missiuna, C., Stewart, D., Law, M., & Wilkins, S. [2006]. *The McMaster Lens for Occupational Therapists*. Hamilton, Ontario, Canada: McMaster University.)

occupational therapist, will have substantial information with which to choose a relevant theoretical approach for assessment, treatment, and evaluation of outcomes after therapy intervention.

Occupational therapists use relevant theoretical approaches to help understand and address the youth's occupational performance issues. Theoretical approaches help therapists understand youth and their chosen occupations, determine why they are encountering issues with specific occupations, and help to guide the process of change (McColl et al., 2003). Theoretical approaches guide the thinking and reasoning of the therapist as he or she selects the most appropriate approach(es) to address a specific occupational performance issue. The term *frame of reference* is conceptually similar to *theoretical approach*, as they both address specific areas of occupation (rather than occupation on its own) to guide occupational therapists in applying theory to specific practice situations (Cole & Tufano, 2008).

McColl et al. (2003) identified five categories of theoretical approaches that are used by occupational therapists. Each theoretical approach is a category that can contain more than one conceptual and/or practice model. It is important to remember that the categories are not, in themselves, models or theories. The theoretical approach categories are represented by the five tabs on the lens (Figure 2-7):

1. Physical—Ways of thinking about the physical determinants of occupation (e.g., muscle strength, range of motion, endurance, and pain)
2. Psychological-emotional—Ways of thinking about the psychological and emotional determinants of occupation (e.g., thoughts and feelings)
3. Cognitive-neurological—Ways of thinking about the cognitive and neurological determinants of occupation (e.g., intellectual ability, sensory processes, and perceptual skills)
4. Sociocultural—Ways of thinking about the social and cultural determinants of occupation (e.g., beliefs, attitudes, roles, and values)
5. Environmental—Ways of thinking about the environmental determinants of occupation (e.g., physical, institutional, economic, legal, political, social, and cultural)

Some examples of theoretical approaches/frames of reference for each category described above are provided in Table 2-1.

As an occupational therapist, the following question is important for your consideration as part of the Theoretical Approach Lens:

1. What theoretical approach(es)/frame(s) of reference and/or model(s) will you use to guide the assessment process?

Table 2-1.

Examples of Theoretical Approaches

Determinants of Occupational Function/Dysfunction (Practice models may also be referred to as frames of reference)	Physical	Psychological-Emotional	Cognitive-Neurological	Sociocultural	Environmental
Conceptual and practice models	Rehabilitative	Cognitive-behavioral therapy	Contemporary task-oriented approach	Temporal adaptation	Ecology of human performance
	Biomechanical	Model of human occupation	Motor learning/control	Model of human occupation	Compensatory (adapt environment, assistive technology)
		Psychiatric rehabilitation	Cognitive rehabilitation	Social competence models	Environmental press
			Dynamic interactional model		
			Sensory processing		

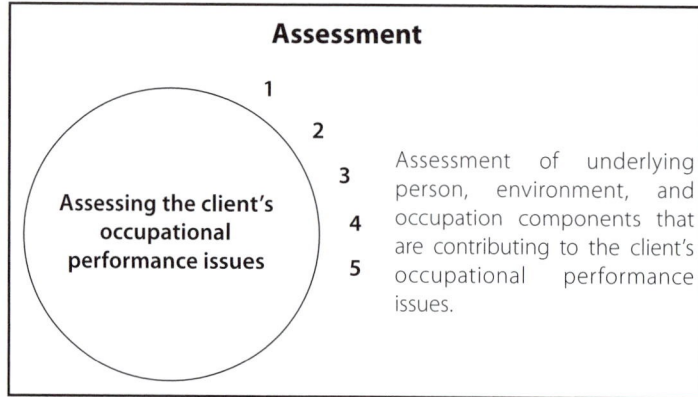

Assessment

Assessing the client's occupational performance issues

1
2
3
4
5

Assessment of underlying person, environment, and occupation components that are contributing to the client's occupational performance issues.

Figure 2-8. The Assessment Lens. (Reprinted with permission from Salvatori, P., Jung, B., Missiuna, C., Stewart, D., Law, M., & Wilkins, S. [2006]. *The McMaster Lens for Occupational Therapists.* Hamilton, Ontario, Canada: McMaster University.)

Consider the fit/lack of fit among the underlying PEO factors in relation to the occupational performance issues when selecting a theoretical approach(es).

Lens #6—Practice Scenario

The practice scenario that we are considering in this chapter is a population-based scenario. The choice of the appropriate theoretical approaches will depend on the nature of the issues experienced by youth in Community A and the therapist's analysis of fit/lack of fit between the youth, the community environment, and the leisure occupations. In general, the occupational therapist does not base his or her theoretical approach on diagnosis or type of disability alone. Research indicates that diagnosis is not a significant predictor of participation for children and youth with physical disabilities (Law et al., 2004). The occupational therapist maintains a flexible approach to the identification of theory to guide the assessment and treatment process. For example, youth with lifelong physical disabilities may be most concerned about social relationships and not about physical issues. The lack of fit with their social environment could guide the therapist to select a sociocultural approach. Also, the lack of supports in the city's current community services for youth with disabilities could suggest an environmental approach to assessment and intervention. Often, the complexity of a situation, such as in this practice scenario, leads the occupational therapist to select more than one theoretical approach.

Lens #6—Assessment

In the Assessment component of the Lens (Figure 2-8) the occupational therapist chooses and implements assessment strategies to gather data concerning the PEO factors that are supporting or hindering the occupational performance issues of concern to the youth and his or her family.

Using the five theoretical approaches put forward by McColl et al. (2003), the assessment process can also be organized according to the five tabs on the lens. This process is described as follows:

1. Physical—Assessment of the physical determinants of occupation (e.g., strength, range of motion, endurance, and mobility)

2. Psychological-emotional—Assessment of the psychological-emotional determinants of occupation (e.g., thoughts, feelings, attitudes, motivation, and coping mechanisms)

3. Cognitive-neurological—Assessment of the cognitive-neurological determinants of occupation (e.g., cognitive processes, memory, sensory processes, reflexes, and balance)

4. Sociocultural—Assessment of the sociocultural determinants of occupation (e.g., social roles and habits, cultural values, and beliefs)

5. Environmental—Assessment of the physical, social, cultural, economic, legal, and political aspects of the environment in which the individual's occupations take place (e.g., home environment, workplace environment, community services, societal attitudes, and government policy and funding support)

Through clinical reasoning, the therapist chooses what characteristics to assess and what specific strategies or measurement tools to use. Examples of assessment strategies include observation, home visits, occupational analysis, dynamic assessment through consultation with team members, and interview of youth and/or family members. Specific standardized and/or non-standardized measurement tools include muscle testing, leisure checklists, physical demands analysis, perceptual tests, ADL inventories, and environmental assessments. These assessment tools are used to gather information about the youth's occupational performance components and environmental conditions that help or hinder occupational performance. The choice of the assessment process and specific measurement tools follows the principles of evidence-based practice in considering the reliability, validity, and clinical utility of each strategy.

For the Assessment component of the Lens, the following question is important for the occupational therapist to consider:

1. Based on your selected theoretical approaches, what is your overall assessment plan?

Consider what assessment strategies you might use for data collection purposes (e.g., interview, direct observation, use of standardized measures, and consultation with professional colleagues).

Within this book, each chapter provides specific assessment approaches and strategies. For the population-based example in this chapter, assessment by the occupational therapist focuses on gathering information about the types of leisure occupations in which youth with disabilities in Community A want to participate. Assessment data regarding environmental supports and barriers within communities can be gathered through a literature review of research and through information provided from youth within the specific community. Assessment methods that could be used effectively within this population-based approach include focus groups and/or surveys of youth and their families within the community.

Fine Tuning the Lens

A unique characteristic of the McMaster Lens for Occupational Therapists is the focus on the flexibility of the occupational therapy process through fine tuning. This design characteristic of the Lens has been influenced greatly by the International Classification of Functioning, Disability and Health (ICF) from the World Health Organization (2001). According to the ICF, participation and quality of life is influenced by a person's health condition, body function and structure, activity, and environments. Occupational therapists use theories that guide an assessment of the youth in order to understand the impact that a health condition is having on occupation. However, occupational therapists only rarely target the underlying impairment as the primary focus of intervention. Often, occupational therapy intervention seeks to change occupational performance through altering the task and/or the environment. A focus on changing the task or environment means that the theories selected to guide the assessment process are congruent with, but not always the same as, the theories that guide intervention.

In the McMaster Lens for Occupational Therapists, the stage of re-examining the theories that were selected is represented by the fine tuning knob. Once the therapist completes an assessment and determines the reason(s) underlying an occupational performance issue, he or she will "fine tune" the theoretical approach to determine the most suitable approach to guide treatment.

After fine tuning, consider the following:

1. Were the selected theoretical approaches useful in explaining the client's occupational performance issues?

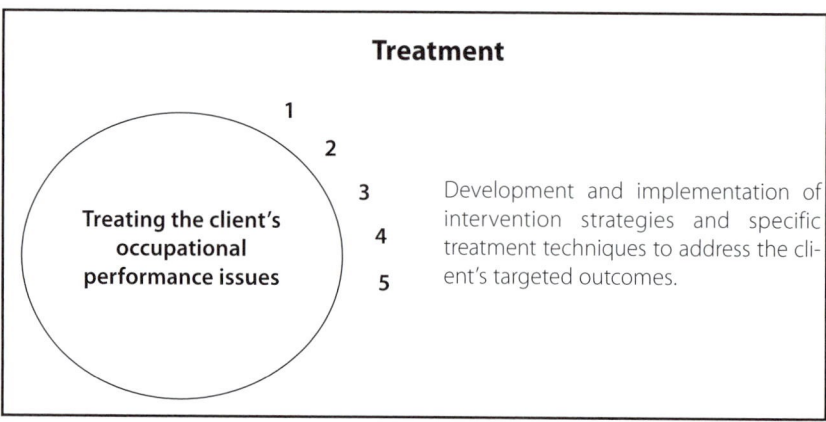

Treatment

1
2
3
4
5

Treating the client's occupational performance issues

Development and implementation of intervention strategies and specific treatment techniques to address the client's targeted outcomes.

Figure 2-9. The Treatment Lens. (Reprinted with permission from Salvatori, P., Jung, B., Missiuna, C., Stewart, D., Law, M., & Wilkins, S. [2006]. *The McMaster Lens for Occupational Therapists.* Hamilton, Ontarior, Canada: McMaster University.)

If yes, then develop an intervention plan that is consistent with the chosen theoretical approach(es). If no, then consider whether you need to select another theoretical approach for intervention or to conduct further assessment of the client's occupational performance issues.

Lens #7—Practice Scenario

Data from a survey of youth in Community A indicate that youth with lifelong disabilities wish to participate in a range of recreation, culture, and sport occupations. The most frequent supports to participation are the availability of a support person, provision of adequate information, and physical accessibility. The most frequent barriers include lack of physical access, lack of information, and poor attitudes of persons working within leisure programs. The occupational therapist analyzes this information and finds that the physical, sociocultural, and environmental theoretical approaches appear to be most appropriate for addressing issues within this community.

Lens #7—Treatment

At Lens #7 (Figure 2-9), the occupational therapist, together with the youth and his or her family, select and implement specific intervention strategies and treatment techniques to address the occupational performance issues. The occupational therapist, at this stage, has selected the most appropriate theoretical approach(es) to guide the intervention process. Working with the youth and his or her family, the specific goals and outcomes of therapy are discussed and agreed upon. Occupational therapy intervention may include strategies to develop, restore, maintain, or promote occupational performance or to prevent occupational dysfunction (CAOT, 1997). In designing intervention strategies, therapists again use the principles of evidence-based practice to select the strategies that are most appropriate for the client, based on his or her needs and evidence of effectiveness demonstrated through research.

In Lens #7, the five categories from McColl et al. (2003) are again used to organize treatment strategies. The occupational therapist implements treatment that is consistent with the five categories of theoretical approaches, as follows:

1.　Physical—Use of physical activity and modalities to address the individual's physical deficits (e.g., strengthening activities, endurance training, activity hardening, and pacing and energy conservation)

2.　Psychological-emotional—Use of approaches to address psychological barriers to occupational performance (e.g., counseling, group therapy, and cognitive behavioral therapy)

3. Cognitive-neurological—Use of approaches that facilitate the restoration of cognitive-neurological capabilities (e.g., cognitive rehabilitation, constraint-induced movement therapy, and sensory processing)

4. Sociocultural—Use of approaches to help the individual rationalize expectations, demands, and restrictive roles and improve relationships with others (e.g., social skills training and group therapy)

5. Environmental—Use of approaches to alter the environment (versus the individual) to improve occupational performance (e.g., removing architectural barriers, job modification, family education, public education, advocacy, and lobbying)

For the Treatment component of the Lens, the following question is considered by the occupational therapist:

1. What is your overall intervention plan?

Consider the occupational therapy role (e.g., direct service, education, consultation, referral, mediator training, and advocacy) and identify specific intervention strategies.

Lens #8—Practice Scenario

Within this book, each chapter provides specific intervention strategies. For all occupational therapy interventions in the area of adult transitions, there are several principles that are followed. Occupational therapy for youth in transition should be occupation based, developmentally appropriate, contextually relevant, evidence based, and client centered. In our specific practice scenario, occupational therapy intervention within Community A can include the following strategies:

» Work together with the city council and community organizations to develop access to a leisure policy for the community.

» Conduct environmental assessments for community recreation, culture and sport organizations, and buildings to determine accessibility and make recommendations for change. Accessibility assessment would focus on physical, information, support, and attitude accessibility.

» Initiate a youth leisure council to provide ongoing advice to the city and community organizations regarding access to leisure occupations.

Lens #8—Outcome

The final Lens (Figure 2-10) focuses on the outcomes of occupational therapy intervention. As treatment progresses, the occupational therapist, youth, and family continually monitor progress and periodically evaluate achievement of the desired occupational performance outcomes. The outcomes of therapy intervention are typically measured in terms of changes in occupational performance, community integration, and participation.

In measuring outcomes after occupational therapy intervention, appropriate measurement strategies and tools are selected to assess changes in the occupational performance issues identified by the youth and his or her family. In some situations, the occupational therapist will use qualitative interviews or structured clinical observations to measure changes in participation/occupational performance. Measurement tools that are reliable and valid and focus at the level of occupation categories such as self-care, productivity, and leisure are selected by many occupational therapists at the end of intervention. In many situations, the assessment of outcomes uses the same tools that were used to identify initial occupational performance issues. For example, if the COPM was used to identify occupational performance issues by the youth, reassessment of outcomes after therapy intervention can use that same measurement tool.

There are very few outcome measures that focus on adult transitions for youth with disabilities in a holistic way. Subsequent chapters of this book describe outcome measurement tools and strategies for specific transition domains. We are beginning to see the development of relevant

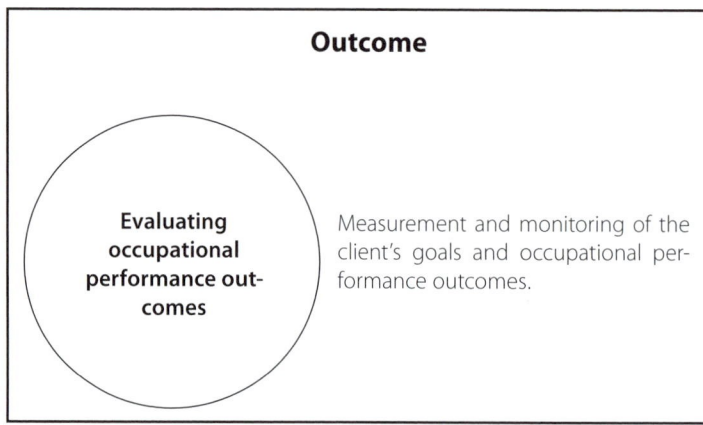

Figure 2-10. The Outcome Lens. (Reprinted with permission from Salvatori, P., Jung, B., Missiuna, C., Stewart, D., Law, M., & Wilkins, S. [2006]. *The McMaster Lens for Occupational Therapists.* Hamilton, Ontario, Canada: McMaster University.)

and developmentally appropriate measures of adult transitions such as the Rotterdam Transition Profile (Wiegerink, Donkervoort, & Roebroeck, 2002) for youth with cerebral palsy, the Self-Management Skills Assessment Guide (Williams et al., 2010), and the TRAQ transition readiness questionnaire (Sawcki et al., 2009) for youth with special health care needs. However, more research and development is needed in this area.

The following question is used by the occupational therapist for the Outcome component of the Lens:

1.   How will you determine if intervention/treatment has been successful?

Consider how you will measure change in occupational performance and client satisfaction.

Practice Scenario

Once the community-based intervention has been completed, the youth leisure council, together with city council and/or community organizations, can conduct satisfaction surveys with youth participating in leisure occupations within Community A. Data from the surveys will provide information regarding satisfaction with participation and can indicate areas for additional access strategies.

Conclusion

This chapter has described the McMaster Lens for Occupational Therapists as a tool to guide therapists in moving theory into practice. Through the use of the Lens, occupational therapists can frame their therapy assessment and intervention for youth in a way that recognizes the complexity of participation in occupations. All relevant perspectives for each youth and his or her families are considered through this process. The lens is flexible and can be used in a bi-directional manner, operating in a forward and reverse direction to understand and assimilate information in guiding the therapeutic process.

Review Questions

1. What is the telescope "metaphor," and how does it connect to occupational therapy practice and values?

2. What is the first lens?

3. What does PEO stand for?

4. How do our roles as occupational therapists make us well-suited to assist youth with disabilities in their transitions to post-secondary education?

References

American Occupational Therapy Association (AOTA). (2008). *Occupational therapy practice framework: Domain and process* (2nd ed.). Bethesda, MD: American Occupational Therapy Association Press.

Canadian Association of Occupational Therapists (CAOT). (1997). *Enabling occupation: An occupational therapy perspective*. Ottawa, Ontario, Canada: CAOT Publication ACE.

Case-Smith, J., Law, M., Missiuna, C., Pollock, N., & Stewart, D. (2010). Foundations for occupational therapy practice with children. In J. Case-Smith & M. O'Brien (Eds.). *Occupational therapy for children* (6th ed.). Maryland Heights, MO: Mosby Elsevier.

Christiansen, C., Baum, C. M., & Bass-Haugen, J. (Eds.). (2005). *Occupational therapy: Performance, participation, and well-being* (3rd ed.). Thorofare, NJ: SLACK Incorporated.

Cole, M. B., & Tufano, R. (2008). *Applied theories in occupational therapy. A practical approach*. Thorofare, NJ: SLACK Incorporated.

Coster, W. J., Deeney, T., Haltiwanger, J., & Haley, S. M. (1998). *School function assessment*. San Antonio, TX: PsychCorp.

Crepeau, E. B., Cohn, E. S., & Boyt Schell, B. A. (Eds.). (2009). *Willard and Spackman's occupational therapy* (11th ed.). New York, NY: Lippincott Williams & Wilkins.

Dunn, W., Brown, C., & McGuigan, A. (1994). The ecology of human performance: A framework for considering the impact of context. *American Journal of Occupational Therapy, 48*(7), 595-607.

Fidler, G. S. (1996). Life-style performance: From profile to conceptual model. *American Journal of Occupational Therapy, 50*(2), 139-147.

Fougeyrollas, P., Noreau, L., & Lepage, (2003). *LIFE-H for children* (pp. 5-13), 1.0. Quebec: INDCP. Retrieved February 15, 2012 from www.ripph.qc.ca/documents/MHAVIE_5-13_ABREGE_AN_repro-interdite.pdf

Janus, A. L. (2009). Disability and the transition to adulthood. *Social Forces, 88*(1), 99-120.

Kielhofner, G. (2008). *A model of human occupation theory and application* (4th ed.). Baltimore, MD: Lippincott Williams & Wilkins.

Kielhofner, G., Mallinson, T., Crawford, C., Nowak, M., Rigby, M., Henry, A., & Walens, D. (2004). *Occupational performance history interview II (OPHI-II) Version 2.1*. Retrieved from www.uic.edu/depts/moho/assess/ophi%202.1.html

Kielhofner, G., Mallinson, T., Forsyth, K., & Lai, J. S. (2001). Psychometric properties of the second version of the occupational performance history interview (OPHI-II). *American Journal of Occupational Therapy, 55*(3), 260-267.

King, G., Law, M., Hanna, S., King, S., Hurley, P., & Rosenbaum, P. (2006). Predictors of the leisure and recreation participation of children with physical disabilities: A structural equation modeling analysis. *Children's Health Care, 35*(3), 209-234.

King, G., Law, M., King, S., Hurley, P., Rosenbaum, P., Hanna, S.,...Young, N. (2004). *Children's assessment of participation and enjoyment (CAPE) and preferences for activities of children (PAC)*. San Antonio, TX: PsychCorp.

Kiresuk, T. J., Smith, A., & Cardillo, J. P. (1994). *Goal attainment scaling: Application, theory and measurement*. Hillsdale, NJ: Lawrence Erlbaum Associates.

Law, M. (Ed.). (1998). *Client-centred occupational therapy*. Thorofare, NJ: SLACK Incorporated.

Law, M., Baptiste, S., Carswell, A., McColl, M. A., Polatajko, H. J., & Pollock, N. (2005). *Canadian Occupational Performance Measure* (4th ed.). Ottawa, Ontario, Canada: CAOT Publications Ace.

Law, M., Cooper, B., Strong, S., Stewart, D., Rigby, P., & Letts, L. (1996). The person-environment-occupation model: A transactive approach to occupational therapy. *Canadian Journal of Occupational Therapy, 63*(1), 9-23.

Law, M., Finkelman, S., Hurley, P., Rosenbaum, P., King, S., King, G., & Hanna, S. (2004). The participation of children with physical disabilities: Relationships with diagnosis, physical function, and demographic variables. *Scandanavian Journal of Occupational Therapy, 11*(4), 156-162.

Mackie, P. C., Jessen, E. C., & Jarvis, S. N. (1998). The lifestyle assessment questionnaire: An instrument to measure the impact of disability on the lives of children with cerebral palsy and their families. *Child: Care, Health, and Development, 24*(6), 473-486.

Mattingly, C., & Fleming, M. (1994). *Forms of inquiry in a therapeutic practice*. Philadelphia, PA: F. A. Davis.

McColl, M. A. (2003). *Spirituality and occupational therapy*. Ottawa, ON: CAOT Publication ACE.

McColl, M.A. (2011). *Spirituality and occupational therapy* (2nd ed.). Ottawa, Ontario, Canada: CAOT Publications ACE.

McColl, M. A., Law, M., Stewart, D., Doubt, L., Pollock, N., & Krupa, T. (2003). *Theoretical basis of occupational therapy* (2nd ed.). Thorofare, NJ: SLACK Incorporated.

Merriam-Webster's Online Dictionary. (2005). Retrieved May 28, 2006 from www.Merriam-webster.com.

Noreau, L., Fougeyrollas, P., Vincent, C. (2002). The LIFE-H: Assessment of the quality of social participation. *Technology and Disability, 14*(3),113-118.

Noreau, L., Lepage., C., Boissiere, L., Picard, R., Fougeyrollas, P., Mathieu, J.,...Nadeau, L. (2007). Measuring participation in children with disabilities using the Assessment of Life Habits. *Developmental Medicine and Child Neurology, 49*(9), 666-671.

Reed, K. L., & Sanderson, S. N. (1999). *Concepts of occupational therapy* (4th ed.). Baltimore, MD: Lippincott Williams & Wilkins.

Salvatori, P., Jung, B., Missiuna, C., Stewart, D., Law, M., & Wilkins, S. (2006). *The McMaster Lens for Occupational Therapists*. Hamilton, Ontario, Canada: McMaster University.

Sawicki, G. S., Lukens-Bull, K., Yin, X., et al. (2009). Measuring the transition readiness of youth with special healthcare needs: Validation of the TRAQ—Transition Readiness Assessment Questionnaire. *Journal of Pediatric Psychology, 36*(2), 160-171. doi10.1093/jpepsy/jsp128

Stewart, D., Law, M., Young, N., Forhan, M., Healy, H., Burke-Gaffney, J., & Freeman, M. (2008). *Understanding the transitional tensions of youth with disabilities in Canada. Identifying key research gaps. Penultimate report to Human Resources Social Development Canada (HRSDC)*. Hamilton, Ontario, Canada: McMaster University. Unpublished document.

Sumsion, T., & Law, M. (2006). A review of evidence on the conceptual elements informing client-centred practice. *Canadian Journal of Occupational Therapy, 73*(3), 153-162.

Townsend, E. A., & Polatajko, H. J. (2007). *Enabling Occupation II: Advancing an occupational therapy vision for health, well-being, and justice through occupation*. Ottawa, ON: CAOT Publications ACE.

Watson, D. E., & Wilson, S. (2003). *Task analysis: An individual and population approach* (2nd ed.). Bethesda, MD: American Occupational Therapy Association Press.

Wiegerink, D., Donkervoort, M., & Roebroeck, M. (2007). *The Rotterdam Transition Profile, Concept 0.2*. Rotterdam: ErasmusMC. Retrieved February 15, 2012 from www.erasmusmc.nl/Reva/Research/transition/RotterdamTransitionProfilev0.2

Williams, T. S., Sherman, E. M. S., Dunseith, C., Mah, J. K., Blackman, M., Latter, J.,...Thornton, N. (2010). Measurement of medical self-management and transition readiness among Canadian adolescents with special health care needs. *International Journal of Adolescent Health, 3*(4), 527-535.

Wood, D., Reiss, J. G., Ferris, M. E., Edwards, L. R., & Merrick, J. (2010). Transition from pediatric to adult care. *International Journal of Child and Adult Health, 3*(4), 445-447.

World Health Organization (WHO). (2001). *International classification of functioning, disability and health*. Geneva, Switzerland: WHO.

3

Transitions From Parents' Home to Independent Living Arrangements for Youth With Physical Disabilities

Andrea Morrison, BSc, OT Reg (Ont); Karen Margallo, MCISc (OT); and Matt Freeman, MA

This chapter uses a scenario to illustrate how the McMaster Lens for Occupational Therapy guides the clinical reasoning process when working with adolescents who are developing their autonomy and skills for independent living. The scenario is based on Mark, who is 16 years old, and starting to plan for his future. The occupational therapist collaborates with Mark in setting and achieving functional goals (in areas of self-care, productivity, and leisure) that will support his aspirations for his life as an adult. The clinical context will set the stage for the scenario, and the client's perspective will be integrated throughout the discussion of the clinical reasoning process.

Clinical Context

At 18 months of age, Mark was referred by his family doctor to a developmental pediatrician following concerns about his motor development. At the age of 24 months, Mark was formally diagnosed with cerebral palsy (CP), which is described as:

> *A group of permanent disorders of the development of movement and posture, causing activity limitations that are attributed to non-progressive disturbances that occurred in the developing fetal or infant brain. The motor disorders of cerebral palsy are often accompanied by disturbances of sensation, perception, cognition, communication, and behavior, by epilepsy, and by secondary musculoskeletal problems. (Rosenbaum, Paneth, Leviton, Goldstein, & Bax, 2007)*

Mark was referred to occupational therapy and physical therapy services by his developmental pediatrician. Since that time, he has been seen on an outpatient basis through the local children's treatment center that offers center and community-based services to children from birth to

Stewart, D. (Ed.)
Transitions to Adulthood for Youth With Disabilities Through an Occupational Therapy Lens (pp. 47-66).
© 2013 SLACK Incorporated

18 years of age who have physical and/or neurodevelopmental disabilities. Therapists may work with clients and their families either on an individual basis or through group-based therapy.

Introduction: Mark at Age 16

Every day my mother gets me up, gets me dressed, and I go to school. Every so often my parents and I meet with my therapist and hear things like: "Your parents are not going to be around to do your care forever." Truthfully, I understand this, but I feel that it is not something I need to worry about immediately. This is something I have time to think about later on. I am okay with the idea of others doing my care, from my experiences at summer camp, but I like my parents handling my care because then I do not have to worry about schedules and they just know what to do.

I do well at school and I like the idea of going to university, maybe living on my own when I am older. I like hanging out with my friends but do not get out of the house as often as I would like. It would be nice to get a job so I would not have to ask my parents for money all the time, maybe in the summer.

Viewing Mark's Situation Through an Occupational Therapy Lens

Occupation, Spirituality, and Development

There are a number of different occupations embedded in this scenario. Self-care occupations are all important for an individual's daily maintenance and personal care. Although self-care occupations may be considered by some to be relatively simple activities of daily living (ADL), they are prerequisites for a person's participation in everyday experiences at home, school, work, and in the community (James, 2008). The groups of self-care occupations that are referred to as instrumental activities of daily living (IADL) are equally important for future adult independence (Vroman, 2010). These include community mobility, financial management, meal preparation, housework, and shopping.

Mark requires physical assistance for all of these self-care occupations, and this places him in a position of dependency upon others. Occupational therapists and other health care professionals now embrace the concept of *interdependence* to acknowledge that the important outcome of intervention is not necessarily "independence"; rather, facilitating a mutual, respectful relationship between an individual who needs assistance and the person providing that assistance (Stewart et al., 2008). Interdependence has been shown to be a significant predictor of life satisfaction, even more so than self-efficacy (Gooden-Ledbetter, Cole, Maher, & Condeluci, 2007). A critical aspect of interdependence is to ensure that the individual who requires assistance has choice and control over what is done. The phrase "directing your own care" represents the desired outcome of autonomy and self-determination for youth with disabilities who need physical assistance for self-care (Stewart et al., 2009).

The other important occupation to consider in this scenario relates to Mark's future living arrangements. The term *independent living* is used extensively in the literature to describe a range of living arrangements for individuals with special needs. This term should not be confused with the *independent living movement* (DeJong, 1979), which represents a social movement with a goal of better quality of life for people with disabilities.

The process and outcomes for youth with disabilities transitioning to independent living have not received a great deal of attention or study (Lawrence, Alleckson, & Bjorklund, 2010; Leiter & Waugh, 2009). The lack of integrated systems of care, including health and social services, has been identified as a barrier for families trying to find appropriate independent living arrangements for their young adult (Lawrence et al., 2010).

Leiter and Waugh (2009) refer to "residential independence" (p. 522) to describe the developmental marker of leaving home. This recognizes that young adults with disabilities may need support when living on their own in whatever type of living arrangement they choose. The authors acknowledge the interdependence with all family members throughout an individual's transition to living on his or her own. They also identify the level of care assistance required by a young adult to be a significant factor in deciding when to leave home and where to live (Leiter & Waugh, 2009).

In the occupational therapy literature, independent living is often considered within the larger picture of community living and participation (Loukas & Dunn, 2010). Research has shown that youth with disabilities lag behind those without disabilities in terms of residing outside of their parents' homes (Loukas & Dunn, 2010).

At Mark's age, spirituality may focus mainly on the *meaning* that he ascribes to the occupations that are important to him—as an adolescent, social occupation with friends is typically the most meaningful (Vroman, 2010). This can influence how he feels about needing assistance from others for personal occupations, and also about his future living arrangements. The meaning that he ascribes to living on his own and away from his parents' home will influence his motivation to take on personal responsibility for directing his own personal care over time. The therapist should therefore explore this with him.

Developmentally, Mark is a typical adolescent who wants to have more personal freedom; however, he is becoming more dependent on his parents for assistance. It is an expectation at his stage in life that he would want to explore having other people provide this assistance. It is also expected that he would want to begin to look to a future of living away from his parents. Although there is a great deal of complexity inherent in this future for Mark, it is one that is developmentally appropriate and should be facilitated as much as possible.

Viewing Mark's situation through these first three lenses can guide the occupational therapist to explore his self-perceptions about daily occupational performance. The Canadian Occupational Performance Measure (COPM) can be used during the initial visit with a client, such as Mark, as it is an individualized, client-centered measure that looks at change in a client's self-perception of occupational performance over time (Law et al., 2005). This assessment provides an overview of the client's priorities, based on level of importance assigned by the client, that relates to the meaning he or she ascribes to different occupations. Table 3-1 provides Mark's COPM scores that will serve as part of the foundation for setting and achieving his functional goals.

For adolescents transitioning to adult living, it is also beneficial to explore their aspirations and vision for the future, as this too will influence his or her own developmental expectations and the meaning they ascribe to different occupations. Clinical interview and anecdotal information can provide a great deal of information regarding goals and priorities. During the initial visit, Mark spoke about his future.

Mark at 16 Years Old—Vision for the Next Year

I feel like there's this pressure to figure out what I'm going to do after high school. I want to get into university. I'm not sure what kind of career or job I want to have, so it's hard to choose a program just yet. I'm strong in English and social sciences; I don't really care for math or biology and stuff. It's a bit stressful having so many decisions to make, but exciting to have choices at the same time. It's great hanging out with my friends—we've talked about getting a place together when we go to university, but I guess this will depend on where I go. If I go to the local university, my parents want me to live at home, because they say it's cheaper and they can still help with my care. Really, I think they just want to be able to keep an eye on me and know that I'm okay.

Mark at 16 Years Old—Vision for the Next 5 Years

I can see myself living in my own apartment when I'm older. I know that I'll need lots of help to do this, but it's definitely something I want to do. I hope I have a decent paying job, a nice apartment, steady girlfriend, and good friends to hang out with. I'll be able to drink by then (legally) so I'm excited about that!

	Importance	Performance	Satisfaction
Table 3-1. **Results of Mark's Initial Canadian Occupational Performance Measure Scores**			
Self-Care			
1. Mark wants to safely transfer in the home environment.	8	6	6
2. Mark wants to use public transportation.	10	1	0
3. Mark wants to start preparing for future "independent living" arrangements.	6	0	2
Productivity			
1. Mark wants to learn about post-secondary options and available supports.	9	5	5
2. Mark wants to explore job skills and opportunities.	10	0	2
3. Mark wants to participate in meal preparation at home.	9	0	2
4. Mark wants to participate in shopping and financial management at home.	7	2	2
Leisure			
1. Mark wants more opportunities to get together with friends outside of school.	10	2	3

Person-Environment-Occupation Analysis

After reviewing Mark's vision, goals, and occupational performance issues, the occupational therapist can examine the interaction between the components of person, environment, and occupation (PEO)and use this information to guide the planning process.

Person Factors

Mark is 16 years old, is in 11th grade at high school, and has an educational assistant to help him manage his books, note-taking, etc. He is taking a full course load and has an A average in most courses. His school performance indicates that he has above-average cognitive skills. He also presents with strong verbal communication skills. He uses a laptop with speech recognition software at home and school for assignments.

In terms of his physical mobility, Mark uses a power wheelchair for mobility at school and out in the community. He requires custom seating to provide adequate trunk and pelvic support. Mark requires full assistance for transfers and lifting, and he uses a floor lift for transfers at school. Mobility in community is important for all adolescents (Figure 3-1).

Mark reports that he has a positive approach to life and is content with his current living situation and level of participation. He believes that he deserves the right to be an independent adult, access the appropriate supports to live on his own, work, and be an included and contributing member of his community, regardless of his disability. Mark is open to exploring options for independent living and is looking forward to graduating from high school and attending a university.

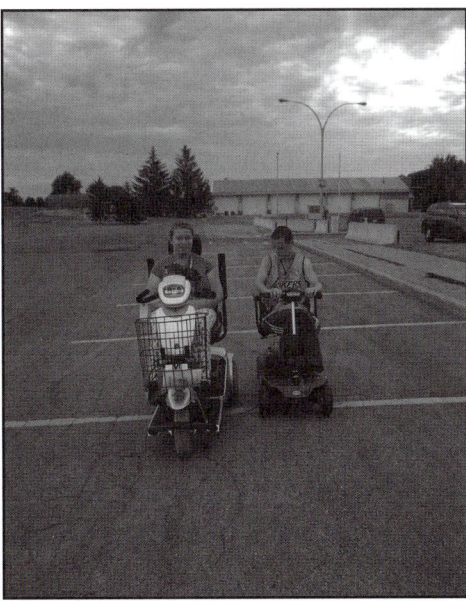

Figure 3-1. Mobility in the community is important for all adolescents.

Environmental Factors

Physical

Mark and his family live in a raised bungalow in a residential neighborhood. He reports that he can get into and out of his house, as his parents have put in ramps, and his bedroom and bathroom are on the main floor. They have not made any other renovations to the house.

Mark lives in an urban city that has an accessible public transit system and specialized wheelchair transit buses. Mark can drive his power wheelchair on most of the sidewalks, as they have cutout curbs, but he cannot go into all stores in his community because of stairs or small door openings. Most of his friends' homes are also inaccessible.

Mark attends his local high school, which is wheelchair accessible with ramps and an elevator to the second floor. The school board provides wheelchair accessible transportation to and from school. Mark also uses a portable floor lift for bathroom transfers. His course schedule has been modified to minimize travel distance between classes. Mark attends therapy sessions on a bi-weekly basis and sees both his physiotherapist and occupational therapist. In terms of transportation, his parents will drive him as their schedules permit; otherwise, he uses the specialized wheelchair transit service.

Social

Mark lives at home with his parents and older sister. His parents have always provided the assistance Mark needs for daily care, including physical transfers. His father works full-time and his mother, part-time. His father recently injured his back when lifting Mark into the bathtub.

Mark has a number of friends and they come to his home after school to play video games or to do homework. He occasionally goes out to the movies with his friends on the weekend, if his parents can drive him. At school, Mark has a full-time educational assistant who goes to all classes with him. She assists him with note-taking, managing books and papers, dressing, and toileting.

Cultural

Mark reports that his family is fairly close and his parents are willing to support him physically. They are a middle-class family, so finances are somewhat limited for post-secondary education and for major home renovations.

The cultural environment also includes the laws and policies surrounding a person. Mark reports that his school has always been inclusive in their approach to his education. He is aware of the special education policies within his high school, but does not know about post-secondary education policies. He is eligible for special equipment funding through the government, but it is a limited amount and he is not sure how this will differ when he becomes an adult.

Occupation Factors

Self-Care

At home, Mark requires physical assistance for all personal care and transfers. His mother does the shopping and most of the housework including meal preparation. He can use his wheelchair to move around in his neighborhood, but relies on his parents to drive him to places in the community, such as movie theaters. His parents control his finances and manage his banking needs. He is not currently sexually active.

Productivity

Mark can do his homework independently using his laptop and speech recognition software. He has said that he would like to find a summer job this year, so he has some money of his own. He is not sure what jobs he could manage and how to go about getting one.

Leisure

Mark's leisure occupations are primarily video games and online conversations with friends. He would like to get together more often with friends, but transportation is not always available. He is an active member of the student council at school and wants to keep this up. He is also interested in pursuing dating but has not yet had a girlfriend.

Analysis

There appears to be a good fit between Mark's social and cognitive skills, the demands of his home and school-based occupations, and current social activities. There is also a good fit between the accessible physical environment and his physical needs for mobility and access. The main concerns at this time are the lack of fit between Mark's need for physical assistance, his developmental stage of expecting independence, and the home environment in which he is dependent on physical assistance. Furthermore, the physical aspects of the home environment are not a good fit for promoting his independence. Mark wants to go away to university, which means that he will be living away from his parents and will need to be able to direct his own care with other people, such as attendants. Ultimately, Mark would like to get his own apartment and therefore needs to develop the knowledge and skills to manage all of the occupations involved in independent living.

Theoretical Approaches

Based on this PEO analysis, the following theoretical approaches to occupational therapy assessment and intervention may be considered. A psychological-emotional approach could assist in exploring aspects of Mark's developing self-efficacy, independence, and autonomy as he transitions to adulthood. A cognitive-neurological approach can be used to address a number of Mark's issues. First, the occupational therapist can focus on his neurological functioning, including muscle tone and coordination, to determine the best strategies for Mark to develop the skills needed to direct his own physical care in daily occupations (e.g., transfers, seating and positioning, bowel/bladder routines, dressing, and showering). A cognitive-neurological approach can also guide the therapist to use a cognitive top-down approach in intervention, to educate Mark about how to plan and execute new tasks, such as learning to direct caregivers in how to transfer him. A sociocultural approach may also be used to explore Mark's changing values and roles, as well as its affect on family dynamics and caregiver roles.

Table 3-2.					
Assessments Used and Their Applicable Theoretical Approach					
Assessment	Physical	Psychological-Emotional	Cognitive-Neurological	Socio Cultural	Environmental
Muscle tone, coordination			X		
GMFCS and MACs				X	X
Home environment assessment	X				X
PSE		X			

An environmental approach will likely be needed to ensure that Mark has the necessary environmental supports and accommodations. This approach will support the therapist's request for a home visit, as a thorough home assessment is needed to make appropriate recommendations to ensure a good person-environment fit. This will enable Mark to participate in the occupations required for future independent living arrangements.

These approaches will be used in parallel as the occupational therapist works to enable optimal occupational performance for Mark as he continues along a developmental trajectory toward independent living. Depending on the results of the assessment and Mark's priorities, the therapist may have to reconsider the theoretical approaches to guide intervention. Table 3-2 shows the link between theoretical approach and assessment.

Assessment

Assessment will focus on exploring the underlying components that are contributing to Mark's current occupational performance issues within the areas of self-care, productivity, and leisure as he identified on the COPM. Clinical interview, observation, and standardized assessments are often used in combination to provide a comprehensive review of the client's needs and to offer direction for intervention and follow-up.

Using a cognitive-neurological approach, the therapist will assess Mark's current neurological functioning. Measurement and observation of muscle tone, coordination, and balance will provide information regarding his physical function as he performs different personal care activities. It is important to assess and monitor changes in range of motion since issues such as joint contractures and pain can arise and limit his functional movement (Katalinic, Harvey, & Herbert, 2011). Motor function can also be classified according to the Gross Motor Functional Classification System—Expanded and Revised (GMFCS—E&R) (Palisano, Rosenbaum, Bartlett, & Livingston, 2007). The GMFCS is helpful in describing a child or youth's present abilities and limitations in gross motor function according to levels (I through V) and by age band (Palisano et al., 2007). The Manual Abilities Classification System (MACS) offers a descriptive approach by level (I through V) related to a child's ability to handle objects in daily activities (Eliasson et al., 2006). By observing the client's motor function, including transfer skills and use of current equipment, the occupational therapist can gain more insight into the level of supports that may be required.

Mark's gross motor function falls within GMFCS Level IV described as the following (Palisano et al., 2007):

> *Youth use wheeled mobility in most settings. Youth require adaptive seating for pelvic and trunk control. Physical assistance from 1 or 2 persons is required for transfers. Youth may support weight with their legs to assist with standing transfers. Indoors, youth may walk short distances with physical assistance, use wheeled mobility, or, when positioned, use a body support walker. Youth are physically capable of operating a powered wheelchair. When a powered wheelchair is not feasible or available, youth are*

transported in a manual wheelchair. Limitations in mobility necessitate adaptations to enable participation in physical activities and sports, including physical assistance and/ or powered mobility.

In terms of the MACS, Mark falls within Level III, which refers to a person who handles objects with some difficulty and slow speed and needs help with many activities (Eliasson et al., 2006). He has increased tone in his hands, with his left being more affected than his right. He is right hand dominant, which he uses for daily activities such as self-feeding, driving his power wheelchair, writing, and typing. As indicated above in the PEO analysis, he requires full support for transfers and lifting.

Application of a psychological-emotional approach for assessment is also appropriate for this scenario. An assessment can be done informally through client interview regarding thoughts, feelings, attitudes, motivation, and coping mechanisms. A formal measure such as the Perceived Self-Efficacy Measure (PSE) can be used to look at change in a client's self-perception of self-efficacy in occupational performance over time and is specifically designed for the adolescent population (Passmore, 2004). *Self-efficacy* is defined as "the belief in one's effectiveness in performing a specific task" (Zimmerman & Cleary, 2006, p. 45) and is considered a key component in one's transition to adulthood. By exploring Mark's level of self-efficacy, we learn that Mark is keen to develop his level of independence and autonomy but is unsure of his abilities when faced with new and unfamiliar situations.

Using an environmental approach to guide assessment, the occupational therapist can consider various aspects including the client's physical, social, and cultural surroundings to determine the supports and/or barriers that may exist. Assessment of the physical environment includes the structure and layout of a space, but also it is most helpful to observe how the youth functions within that space. The social environment includes family, friends, and other people within the youth's network of support. Cultural factors may include the various programs or services that the youth currently accesses or might access in future, as well as financial support, and local and macro-level government policies and regulations. These cultural factors reflect the beliefs, moral values, traditions, language, and laws that influence a young person in transition to adult life.

A thorough assessment of Mark's home is necessary for intervention planning. The physical assessment of Mark's home reveals that it has been renovated in parts by his parents, to accommodate the use of a power wheelchair. There is a ramp into the house from the garage, and his bedroom is on the main floor. His kitchen is small and not set up for wheelchair access (e.g., counter tops are standard height). He has wheelchair access to the bathroom, which contains a standard tub, vanity sink, and toilet. There is a ceiling track system installed for transfers to/from the tub and toilet; however, his parents have not been using the lift as part of his daily routines.

Mark is surrounded by family and friends who are accepting and supporting of his needs. Financially, Mark's family is receiving a monthly income benefit from the government, which provides financial support for some medical, dental, and equipment needs. Given Mark's diagnosis and the family income, he is also eligible to receive financial subsidy/supports for transportation and education.

Fine Tuning

Upon review of the assessment findings, no changes were necessary in terms of the three theoretical approaches that were guiding the occupational therapist's reasoning. These continued to be appropriate approaches for intervention.

Intervention

It is important to prioritize and discuss treatment goals with the client and negotiate the desired outcomes. Setting goals and therapy objectives in conjunction with the client is essential for engaging the client in the therapeutic process. Therapy objectives should be written as SMART goals so that the client and therapist have a clear understanding of what is expected (Doran, 1981). SMART refers to goals that are: specific (S), measurable (M), achievable (A), realistic (R), and time oriented (T). Action plans provide a detailed description on how clients' goals will be achieved.

In reviewing the COPM results, Mark has prioritized the following goal areas:

» To use public transportation.

» To apply for a job.

» To go on a community outing together with friends outside of school.

» To plan and prepare a meal.

» To direct caregivers in the use of safe transfer routines.

Mark was given the option to address these goals in one-on-one therapy sessions and/or a group format. He indicated a preference to do a combined approach to achieve his goals. Mark was informed about teen groups offered through the children's treatment center, such as a cooking group, Independent Living Skills Program (ILSP), a public transportation group, and the Youth Advisory Committee, which plans social events for youth and gives youth input into programming. Mark indicated that he was busy with school and student council activities and would prefer to participate in a summer program targeting independent living skills. He also expressed an interest in joining the Youth Advisory Committee.

Individual Direct Therapy

Goal: To Use Public Transportation

The occupational therapist starts with the client's current ability to read maps and bus schedules, plan a bus route (with direct and transfer options), and wheelchair mobility skills. When working with a client to use public transportation, the occupational therapist may want to consider the following aspects: travel routes, fare costs, boarding and de-boarding sites, demonstration of pedestrian skills necessary for travel route, communication/social skills in public places, and problem solving for unexpected situations (e.g., getting lost, missing a stop, or wheelchair breaking down). The occupational therapist may suggest riding the bus together several times so that any challenges in using public transportation can be identified and hopefully solved together.

Mark lives in a suburban neighborhood with easy access to public transportation. All buses in the city have an accessible low floor for wheelchair access. He was on the bus before with his older sister but did not participate in planning the trip and is nervous about going on the bus on his own. He can use his excellent skills in navigating the Internet and looking up bus schedules. Ultimately, Mark would like to be able to take the bus so that he can meet up with his friends in the community.

Therapy Objectives and Timelines Are Negotiated With Mark to Guide the Treatment Process

1. Within 1 week, Mark will plan a round-trip bus route from his house to the movie theater so that he can watch an evening show.

2. Within 2 months, Mark will use public transportation with minimal occupational therapist support and practice bus travel on this route a minimum of two times.

3. Mark will use public transportation to travel independently to/from the movie theater within 3 months.

Goal: To Develop Job Search Skills

Since there are many factors for persons with disabilities to consider when searching for a job, the occupational therapist can help the client identify the key factors in ensuring a good fit between person, job, and environment. The occupational therapist and client can work together to identify areas for skill training or potential modifications to job tasks and/or work environment. The occupational therapist can also assist the client in identifying his or her skills and creating a resumé to reflect his or her strengths and abilities. Therapeutic techniques such as role-playing and relaxation training can help develop skills such as interviewing, assertiveness, and the ability to deal with stressful situations.

Mark is motivated to obtain a job and has volunteer experience on his student council. He has no idea of what kinds of jobs would be suitable given his abilities or what type of job he would like to pursue.

Therapy Objectives and Timelines

1.　Within 1 month, Mark will develop a draft of a resumé.

2.　Within 2 months, Mark will visit a community agency, which provides job postings, job search tools, and interview preparation strategies.

3.　Within 3 months, Mark will apply for a job that he feels is a good match for his abilities and interests.

Goal: To Go on a Community Outing Together With Friends Outside of School Hours

The occupational therapist can assist the client in exploring community options that are a good fit with his or her interests, as well as consider other factors such as scheduling, cost, accessibility, and supports available. If available, a referral to therapeutic recreation may also be considered.

Mark is socially active at school but finds it challenging to get together with friends outside of school hours. Currently, Mark is dependent on availability of transportation from his parents or the specialized transportation service that requires pre-booking. Mark is developing his skills in using public transportation so that he can meet up with friends more spontaneously. He also needs to consider the accessibility of the location where he will meet with his friends.

Therapy Objectives and Timelines

1.　Within the next month, Mark will identify five community activities in which he and his friends would be interested in participating.

2.　Within 3 months, Mark will independently make arrangements (including travel) and attend an outing with his friends.

Goal: To Plan and Prepare a Meal

The occupational therapist uses occupational analysis skills and clinical reasoning to explore the subjective experience for Mark in learning to prepare a meal. The performance demands of meal preparation in his home environment must be weighed against his own personal abilities and interests. The results of an occupational analysis will guide the therapist to determine whether individual skills can be further developed or if modifications are required. There are 2 types of modifications that can be considered: (1) environmental and (2) task adaptation. An environmental approach will definitely guide part of this treatment plan, as there are several basic environmental modifications that could assist Mark. These include physical modifications, such as relocating items so they are stored within the client's reach, separate preparation area at a height that Mark can reach, and an angled mirror over the preparation and cooking area for better visibility. There will also be the need for some modifications to the social environment, with a focus on helping Mark's mother reduce the amount of assistance and preparation that she provides. The amount and type of assistance can be graded over time as Mark learns new skills and gains confidence.

Task adaptation refers to altering the method and/or tool (Figure 3-2). For example, a microwave or toaster oven could be used in place of the stove top and/or oven. Other ways of cooking include using an electric frying pan or hot plate that could be placed on a lower surface for Mark to use. Ergonomic handles provide easier grip and positioning while using kitchen utensils. Mark

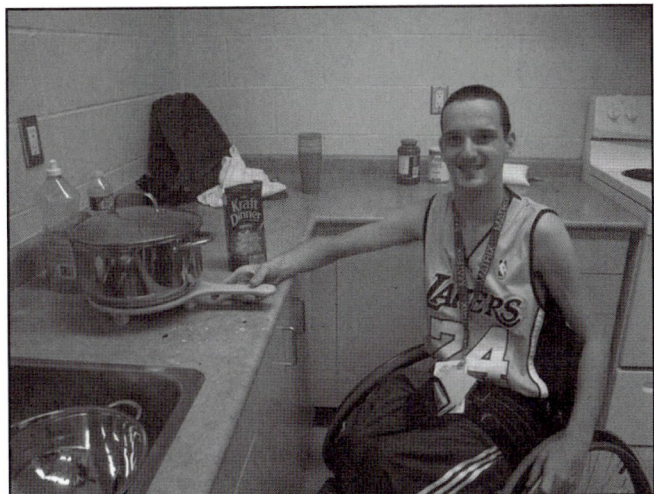

Figure 3-2. Meal planning can require environmental and task adaptation to enable occupational performance.

requires unilateral cooking tools, such as an adaptive cutting board, mounted jar opener, pot stabilizer, and one-handed electric can opener. Being able to direct someone else to prepare a meal in a way that suits a client's preferences also falls within task adaptation. The intervention strategies for this will involve Mark and his parents. Mark will need to learn how to direct his mother to assist him in the kitchen in a respectful but assertive manner, and his mother will need to learn how to wait for Mark to direct her to do something instead of automatically doing it herself. This change in their relationship will take time and patience, and the occupational therapist can support them through this process.

Mark would like to start by preparing a simple meal, such as making a sandwich for lunch. Given Mark's increased muscle tone and limited range of motion, bi-manual kitchen tasks are difficult, such as cutting with a knife, using a can opener, stirring items in a pot/bowl, and peeling fruits and vegetables. The kitchen counters and cupboards are at the standard height and not wheelchair accessible, which limits Mark's ability to accomplish tasks such as cooking on the stove. The family has indicated that they are not in a position to make major modifications to the kitchen. However, Mark's parents are willing to purchase small appliances and kitchen aids.

Mark recognizes that in the long term, if he wants to live in a residence or a supported living apartment, he must become better able to direct others on how he would like a meal prepared. Even cooking a simple meal can be a lengthy process when multiple adaptations are required. Mark will need to find a balance between how much time and energy he wants to exert in preparing a meal versus how much support he can request from his caregivers and/or attendant support workers.

Therapy Objectives and Timelines

1. Within 1 week, Mark and his mother will discuss options for relocating equipment and food items in a cupboard that he can access.

2. Mark will obtain an adaptive cutting board and one-handed electric can opener within 1 week.

3. Mark will independently prepare a simple meal using the microwave and/or toaster oven within 1 month.

4. Mark will provide step-by-step direction to his caregiver(s) on how to prepare a desired meal within 3 months.

Goal: To Direct Caregivers in the Use of Safe Transfer Routines

The occupational therapist reviews, instructs, and provides training to the client and his or her caregiver(s) on the safe use of the lift/transfer equipment. The review includes ensuring the appropriate sizing and design of a sling to provide adequate support during lifts/transfers. In training the use of a lift system, the occupational therapist should consider factors such as client/caregiver readiness, learning ability and style, format for instruction, and schedule of maintenance.

The action plans for this goal will be guided mostly by an environmental approach. Within the physical environment, Mark has an existing ceiling track lift system in his home that is not currently being used. The lack of use is primarily related to the social environment at home. In the past, his father felt it was faster to just lift and carry him; however, with his back injury, he is no longer able to do this. No other caregivers can physically lift Mark and, therefore, they need to learn how to use the lift. Looking to the future, it is most appropriate for Mark to participate in developing step-by-step instructions for using the lift system so that he can direct his parents and future support staff.

Therapy Objective and Timeline

1. Mark will provide step-by-step direction to his parents on proper use of the ceiling track lift system to transfer him to/from his bed, wheelchair, and/or commode within 1 week.

Group-Based Intervention

Occupational therapists can play a unique role in developing group programs for youth transitioning to adult living. There is a strong emphasis on developing life skills, fostering autonomy, and increasing participation to prepare youth for independence or interdependence in adulthood (Kingsnorth, Healy, & Macarthur, 2007). Programs targeting life skills often include goal setting, problem solving, decision making, and developing appropriate personal and interpersonal skills (Loukas & Dunn, 2010). Various skills and/or skill sets can be effectively taught in a group setting, such as cooking, using public transportation, money management, and social skills. Given that social occupations are most meaningful to adolescents (Vroman, 2010), group-based therapy often appeals to this age group and allows them an opportunity to connect with peers who may face similar challenges related to their physical disabilities.

Independent Living Skills Program

The following program description provides an example of an ILSP that was designed to meet the needs of a specific population. The participant criteria for the group are not prerequisites or expectations for all types of life skills programs. Clinicians must consider the unique needs of the target population and available resources when developing programs and making decisions regarding participant criteria, program focus, content, and format.

Participant Criteria and Program Focus

This particular ILSP is offered by a multidisciplinary team from Mark's children's treatment center in a community-based setting. The program is designed to assist youth with physical disabilities, between the ages of 14 to 18, to develop independent living skills. Group participants must be interested in learning new skills related to independent living within a group setting. He or she must have the cognitive ability to direct his or her own care and demonstrate problem solving and personal goal-setting skills.

Directing one's care and developing community mobility/integration skills (e.g., use of public transportation and accessibility within the community) are considered key goals of the program. Other examples of living skills that are emphasized include budgeting, time management, meal

Table 3-3.	
Considerations When Developing and Planning Group Programs	
Purpose of program	• Identify purpose and overall goals of group
Participant criteria	• Identify age range of prospective participants
	• Identify skills required to participate in group
	• Indicate minimum and maximum number of participants
Program format	• Length of program
	• Timing
	• Frequency
	• Location
Schedule	• Review and organize content and outcomes, as appropriate
Staffing	• Identify coordinator(s)/contact person for group
	• Recruit appropriate staff/students/volunteers, as per participant requirements and program needs
Evaluation	• Formal and informal measures
	• Arrange for feedback from participants/caregivers for outcome evaluation and quality improvement
	• Arrange feedback from group staff for quality improvement

preparation, social and communication skills, advocacy, and vocational planning. Information will also be shared about housing and attendant care options, managing medical care, and financial resources. In addition, the program serves to increase participants' awareness and exposure to community resources to promote leisure and a healthy lifestyle. Considerations for program development and planning are listed in Table 3-3.

Youth are provided with various skill-building activities and learning sessions to expose them to typical daily activities involved in living independently (e.g., scheduling and directing one's care using an attendant, self-care, and home management tasks). "Teaching" approaches include goal setting, mentorship, group discussions, problem solving, didactic teaching, homework assignments, role-playing, and exposure to real-life situations.

The peer component of programs such as ILSP can help youth to develop both self-reliance and interdependence through increased awareness of shared needs and experiences (Healy & Rigby, 1999). Furthermore, Healy and Rigby (1999) suggest that "learning about other experiences and strategies they [youth with disabilities] have used can help young people with disabilities to build a foundation of knowledge that they can access at any appropriate time" (p. 242). Given Mark's goals of developing his autonomy and independence, he was a suitable candidate for the intensive group summer program, which is run on an outpatient basis. Mark is motivated to participate and has set out specific goals for ILSP.

Program Format and Content

An intensive group program format was offered, since most participants were available over the summer months and were interested in attending a group program. During the first 4 days, the participants only attend camp for the day and then return home at the end of the day. There is a strong emphasis on goal setting and planning during this first week, so the program is individualized for the participant (Figure 3-3). The program sessions introduce the practical aspects of community mobility, money management, and participation. The second week of the program is an intensive residential program, which includes 5 days and 4 nights. The program activities

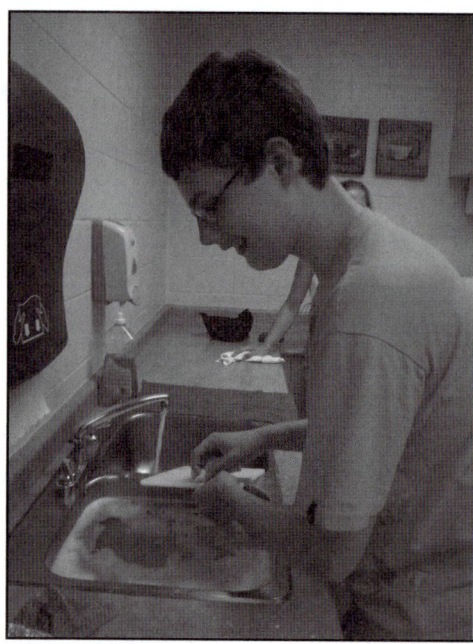

Figure 3-3. The ILSP includes basic home management skills.

promote reinforcement and continued development of skills. The schedule includes "Independent Goal Day," is a day designated for participants to work toward the individualized goals that they set at the beginning of camp.

The ILSP is run by a multidisciplinary team of health care professionals and support staff which include occupational therapists, a therapeutic recreationist, a social worker, physiotherapists, a program assistant, an attendant services coordinator, attendant staff, and volunteers/students. Table 3-4 illustrates a sample schedule of a 9-day ILSP, which includes 4 days of daytime-only programming and a 5-day/4-night residential component.

Prior to ILSP, participants and their caregivers attend an orientation session that outlines the purpose of the program and expectations for participants. Each group member is encouraged to participate in all group sessions, community outings, and fitness activities to the best of his or her ability, seeking assistance from staff as necessary. The importance of maintaining confidentiality within the group is emphasized to create an environment where participants can share their experiences and trust each other. Participants work together in pairs to plan a meal, grocery shop, and prepare the meal. Each participant has a budget for camp and tracks his or her personal expenses while at camp. Community outings are done in small groups with a therapist who assists participants in planning bus routes and taking public transportation. Participants are also responsible for doing their own laundry during the second week of the program.

As previously mentioned, each participant develops several individualized goals that he or she will work toward completing during ILSP, under the direct supervision of program staff.

In conjunction with his occupational therapist, Mark developed the following goals to be accomplished during the 2-week ILSP.

Directing Care

1. Mark will direct an attendant to carry out his shower routine.
2. Mark will direct an attendant to assist with meal preparation (Figure 3-4).

Table 3-4.
Sample Schedule for an Independent Living Skills Program

Week 1

Time	Tuesday	Wednesday	Thursday	Friday
9:00am	Welcome!	Directing your services and booking attendant services	Resumé/job search skills	Bowling
9:30	Goal setting			
10:00			Fitness break	
10:30		Fitness break	Resumé/job search skills	
11:00				
11:30	Bring your own lunch	Bring your own lunch	Bring your own lunch	Lunch—dining out
12:00pm				
12:30	Budgeting for camp	Neighborhood scavenger hunt	Community bussing challenge	
1:00				
1:30	Fitness break	Menu planning		
2:00				
2:30	Transportation	Preparing for bus outings		
3:00			Debrief	Debrief, goal review
3:30	Wrap up and reminders	Goal, budget, and bus review	Goal, budget, and bus review	

Week 2

Time	Monday	Tuesday	Wednesday	Thursday	Friday
8:00am		Morning routine	Morning routine	Morning routine	Morning routine
8:30	Staff briefing	Breakfast and staff briefing/ participant reviews	Breakfast and staff briefing/ participant reviews	Breakfast and staff briefing/ participant reviews	Breakfast and staff briefing/ participant reviews
9:00	Participant welcome and orientation	Visiting housing options in the community	Independent goal day (lunch out in the community)		Packing
9:30					
10:00	Check-in and get settled in rooms			Yoga	Review goals
10:30	Planning for independent goal day and housing visits				
11:00				Goal review	
11:30					Feedback and evaluations
12:00pm	Participants— bring your own lunch			Lunch (including preparation and clean up)	
12:30					Lunch preparation
1:00		Lunch out in community			

(continued)

Table 3-4 (continued).				
Sample Schedule for an Independent Living Skills Program				
Week two				
Time	Monday	Tuesday	Wednesday	Thursday	Friday
1:30pm	Community challenge—grocery shopping	Lunch out in the community	Independent goal day (lunch out in the community)	Laundry	Wrap-up session and parent open house
2:00		Taking charge of your medical care			
2:30				Teen talk—topic set by teens (e.g., bullying, dating, etc.)	
3:00		Planning for goal day			
3:30					
4:00	Community challenge review and feedback			Laundry	
4:30	Dinner (including preparation and clean up)	Dinner (including preparation and clean up)	Dinner (including preparation and clean up)	Dinner (including preparation and clean up)	
5:00					
5:30					
6:00					
6:30					
7:00	Debrief	Debrief	Debrief	Debrief	
7:30					
8:00	Overnight stay	Overnight stay	Overnight stay	Overnight stay	

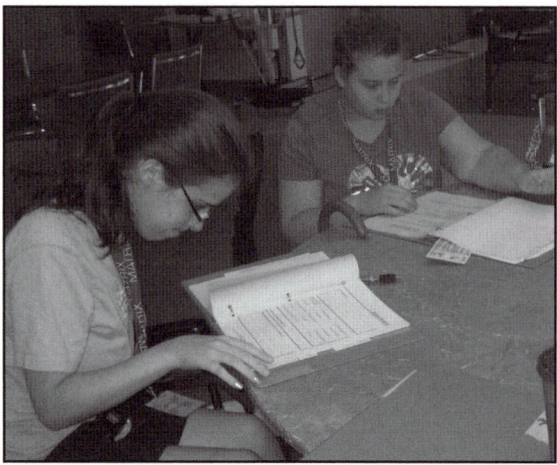

Figure 3-4. The first days of the group program focus on goal setting and planning.

Cooking

1. Mark will make salad and pizza with assistance.
2. Mark will use an adapted cutting board to cut vegetables.

Using Public Transportation

1. Prior to independent goal day, Mark will independently plan the bus route from the camp facility to/from the local university.

2. On independent goal day, Mark will take the bus route to/from the local university with supervision from a therapist.

Exploring Post-Secondary Options

1. On independent goal day, when Mark visits the local university and meets with the Student Services Office, he will inquire about academic programs, residence options, and accessibility services for students.

Independent Living Arrangements

1. Mark will learn about rental and utility costs, the application process, and the waiting list of an assistive living program when he visits an assistive living facility that offers 24-hour attendant care to residents.

Although these may seem like a large number of goals, Mark felt he would be able to achieve them as he was already working on similar goals in the individual treatment sessions with an occupational therapist. The combination of both individual and group intervention allowed Mark to work on multiple goals in a short period of time.

At the conclusion of camp, Mark commented on his experience:

> *Camp was a great experience for me. I loved staying up late hanging out with my new friends. We had lots of laughs and fun on our outings. At first, it was a bit overwhelming figuring out the bus routes, but I was used to it by the end of camp. I felt good when I could help other people plan their bus routes. I also liked being able to do the things I wanted to do—like visit the university and apartments. Now, I can really see myself being there someday and making it on my own. I can't do everything on my own, but I know I can ask others to help me out.*

Outcomes

Evaluation of outcomes is important in establishing the validity of occupational therapy. Re-administration of formal assessments provides pre- and post-quantitative data for comparison. Informal evaluation, such as satisfaction questionnaires and anecdotal reports, provide qualitative data that might not be captured in the numbers. For youth in transition, it is important to keep in mind that new goals may constantly arise, and they may not all be achieved by the time the required discharge and transfer to adult services is required. Transition is a process that can continue well into becoming an adult.

To address Mark's concerns about transition to independent living, individual and group-based therapy goals were set, using the initial findings from the COPM. In re-administering the COPM, only performance and satisfaction are scored (Table 3-5).

A review of the goals that Mark set will provide more anecdotal information related to what he has accomplished. Shortly after attending ILSP, the occupational therapist meets with Mark and his caregivers to review what he has accomplished both at home and at ILSP. Mark reports that he is engaging in more activities at home and in the community with friends. He is using public transportation on a regular basis to get around the community on his own and with friends. He is continuing to practice directing his care for toileting, shower, and meal preparation routines. His parents are making a conscious effort to modify their behavior, such as waiting for him to request assistance or provide instructions regarding his personal care. Time constraints can play a factor in how much they are able to step back and wait for his instruction. He has not yet found a job but is in his final year of high school, so he will be focusing on academics to ensure he has

Table 3-5. Results of Mark's COPM Scores—6 Months Post-Intervention				
	Performance	Difference	Satisfaction	Difference
Self-Care				
1. Mark wants to safely transfer in the home environment	8	+2	8	+2
2. Mark wants to use public transportation	9	+8	10	+10
3. Mark wants to start preparing for future "independent living" arrangements	6	+6	7	+5
Productivity				
1. Mark wants to learn about post-secondary options and available supports	7	+2	7	+2
2. Mark wants to explore job skills and opportunities	7	+7	7	+5
3. Mark wants to participate in meal preparation at home	7	+7	7	+5
4. Mark wants to participate in shopping and financial management at home	5	+3	5	+3
Leisure				
1. Mark wants more opportunities to get together with friends outside of school	9	+7	10	+7

the grades to get into a university. In addition to reviewing previous targeted outcomes, Mark and his caregivers have identified the following new goals:

1. Mark will make his own lunch to take to school.
2. Mark will participate in at least one skill-building group within the next 6 months to continue with skills learned from ILSP.
3. Mark will participate in the next Youth Advisory Committee meeting.
4. Mark will register with Outreach Attendant Services and request attendant services to help him carry out his shower routine at home within the next month.

From a program and organizational perspective, evaluation explores aspects such as program effectiveness, objective achievement, impact, cost-benefit, as well as strategies for improvement. The positive results of the COPM can provide solid evidence of the impact of occupational therapy services, on an individual and group basis. A follow-up client satisfaction survey about the ILSP summer group is conducted each year to show the benefit of this program to a large group of clients. Continual evaluation is required to ensure best practice and quality of services.

Conclusion

Adolescence is a time when youth tend to be very focused on the here and now, juggling the demands of school, family, and relationships with peers. It can be challenging to engage clients and caregivers in the process of planning for the future because there are so many other immediate needs.

There are many aspects of occupational performance related to independent living, including directing your own care, managing activities of daily living and instrumental activities of daily living, living on your own, and being a productive and contributing member of the community. The skill of directing others in your care is a major aspect of managing independent living for a person with a physical disability. It is important for the occupational therapist to explore the balance between time and energy expenditure versus time and energy conservation using supports, such as attendant care. Allowing attendants to assist with certain tasks can free up time and energy to put toward other, more important activities within the day.

Individual therapy allows the youth to focus on personal issues and very specific goals, at his or her own pace. In the ILSP group-based program, youth are given the opportunity to address individual goals, as well as participate with their peers in practical learning experiences to help prepare them for the transition to adult living. When youth learn new skills, it can lead to an increase in their self-esteem and confidence in their abilities, thereby increasing self-efficacy.

Youth are also exposed to a variety of community-based activities and resources that will assist them in planning for their future needs related to such things as housing, transportation, education, vocation, and recreation. Dennis, Williams, Giangreco, and Clonginer (1993) suggest that access to housing, jobs, transportation, and friendships contributes to one's quality of life.

Group-based therapy offers participants the ability to learn and practice new skills in a social and supportive environment with other youth who have similar experiences and face similar barriers to independent living. Youth can learn from each other and gain different perspectives and approaches on how to manage interdependent living.

Directing one's care and participating in group activities fosters interdependence. Gooden-Ledbetter and colleagues (2007) suggest that interdependence and self-efficacy are critical to achieving life satisfaction and, as such, are necessary components of independent living programs.

Occupational therapists provide a unique perspective through which current and future occupations for youth with disabilities can be viewed and explored. They provide a holistic approach to assist youth and their families in looking to the future and planning for interdependent living.

Epilogue—Mark at 30 Years of Age

When I was 16 years old, like the majority of youth with disabilities, my parents were responsible for my personal care. Like other adolescents, this care was something I took for granted. Unfortunately, I had not considered the fact that my parents were aging and performing my care on a regular basis was impacting their health. My transition to attendant care was forced because my mother required knee surgery and my father was working early morning shifts. Following my satisfaction with my attendant services, my occupational therapist began having a conversation with me about moving out of the house and what my future independence would look like. This was a much easier conversation for me to have, since I no longer had the perspective that I could rely on my parents to handle everything. Now I live on my own, in my own apartment in a completely different city than my family. I have attendant services that I use multiple times, daily. I have my routines, my schedules. Most times it all works out; sometimes it doesn't—but you roll with the punches. I see my family when I can. I have my own life now, and it's pretty good.

Review Questions

1. What is the occupation therapist's definition and view of "interdependence" and how does it relate to independent living?

2. What assessments did the occupational therapist implement with Mark around independent living? What approaches guided the type of assessments chosen?

3. What are some considerations for developing and planning a group-based intervention program?

4. What is the purpose and focus of an Independent Living Skills Program (ILSP)? How might it impact youth with physical disabilities? What were some of the outcomes for Mark?

References

DeJong, G. (1979). Independent living: From social movement to analytic paradigm. *Archives of Physical Medicine and Rehabilitation, 60*(10), 435-446.

Dennis, R., Williams, W., Giangreco, M., & Clonginer, C. (1993). Quality of life as context for planning and evaluation of services for people with disabilities. *Exceptional Children, 59*(6), 499-512.

Doran, G. T. (1981). There's a S.M.A.R.T. way to write management's goals and objectives. *Management Review, 70*(11) (AMA Forum), 35-36.

Eliasson, A. C., Krumlinde Sundholm, L., Rösblad, B., Beckung, E., Arner, M., Öhrvall, A. M., Rosenbaum, P. (2006). The Manual Ability Classification System (MACS) for children with cerebral palsy: Scale development and evidence of validity and reliability. *Developmental Medicine and Child Neurology, 48*(7), 549-554.

Gooden-Ledbetter, M. J., Cole, M. T., Maher, J. K., & Condeluci, A. (2007). Self-efficacy and interdependence as predictors of life satisfaction for people with disabilities: Implications for independent living programs. *Journal of Vocational Rehabilitation, 27*(3), 153-161.

Healy, H., & Rigby, P. (1999). Promoting independence for teens and young adults with physical disabilities. *Canadian Journal of Occupational Therapy, 66*(5), 240-249.

James, A. B. (2008). Activities of daily living and instrumental activities of daily living. In E. B. Crepeau, E. S. Cohn, & B. A. Boyt Schell (Eds.), *Willard and Spackman's occupational therapy* (11th ed., pp. 538-578). New York, NY: Lippincott Williams & Wilkins.

Katalinic, O. M., Harvey, L. A., Herbert, R. D. (2011). Effectiveness of stretch for the treatment and prevention of contractures in people with neurological conditions: A systematic review. *Physical Therapy, 91*(1), 11-24.

Kingsnorth, S., Healy H., & Macarthur, C. (2007). Preparing for adulthood: A systematic review of life skill programs for youth with physical disabilities. *Journal of Adolescent Health, 41*(4), 323-332.

Law, M., Baptiste, S., Carswell, A., McColl, M. A., Polatajko, H. J., & Pollock, N. (2005). *Canadian Occupational Performance Measure* (4th ed.). Ottawa, Ontario, Canada: CAOT Publications Ace.

Lawrence, D. H., Alleckson, D. A., & Bjorklund, P. (2010). Beyond the roadblocks: Transition to adulthood with Asperger's disorder. *Archives of Psychiatric Nursing, 24*(4), 227-238.

Leiter, V., & Waugh, A. (2009). Moving out: Residential independence among young adults with disabilities and the role of families. *Marriage and Family Review, 45*, 519-537.

Loukas, K. M., & Dunn, M. L. (2010). Instrumental activities of daily living and community participation. In J. Case-Smith & M. O'Brien (Eds.), *Occupational therapy for children* (6th ed., pp. 518-539). Maryland Heights, MI: Mosby Elsevier.

Palisano, R., Rosenbaum, P., Bartlett, D., & Livingston, M. (2007). *Gross Motor Function Classification System— Expanded and Revised.* Hamilton, ON: CanChild Centre for Childhood Disability Research, McMaster University. Retrieved October 28, 2011 from http://motorgrowth.canchild.ca/en/GMFCS/resources/GMFCS-ER.pdf

Passmore, A. (2004). A measure of perceptions of generalized self-Eefficacy adapted for adolescents. *OTJR: Occupation, Participation and Health, 24*(2), 64-71.

Rosenbaum, P., Paneth, N., Leviton, A., Goldstein, M., & Bax, M. (2007). A report: the definition and classification of cerebral palsy April 2006. *Developmental Medicine and Child Neurology, 49*(s109), 8-14

Stewart, D., Freeman, M., Law, M., Healy, H., Burke-Gaffney, J., Forhan, M., Young, N., & Guenther, S. (2009). *The best journey to adult life for youth with disabilities: An evidence-based model and best practice guidelines for the transition to adulthood for youth with disabilities.* Hamilton, Ontario, Canada: McMaster University.

Stewart, D., Law, M., Young, N., Forhan, M., Healy, H., Burke-Gaffney, J., & Freeman, M. (2008). *Understanding the transitional tensions of youth with disabilities in Canada. Identifying key research gaps. Penultimate report to Human Resources Social Development Canada (HRSDC).* Hamilton, Ontario, Canada: McMaster University. Unpublished document.

Vroman, K. (2010). In transition to adulthood: The occupations and performance skills of adolescents. In J. Case-Smith & J. C. O'Brien (Eds.), *Occupational therapy for children* (6th ed.). St. Louis, MO: Elsevier.

Zimmerman, B., & Cleary, T. (2006). Adolescents' development of personal agency: The role of self-efficacy beliefs and self-regulatory skill. In F. Pajares & T. Urdan (Eds.), *Self efficacy beliefs of adolescents* (pp. 45-69). Greenwich, CT: Age Publishing.

4

Community Participation Through Work Experience for Youth With Developmental Disabilities

*Linda Armour, BSc; Jan Burke-Gaffney; and
Debra Stewart, MSc, OT Reg (Ont)*

This chapter illustrates the importance of active community participation for youth with developmental disabilities. The scenario is a work experience program that provides opportunities for Jesse, a young man with Down syndrome, to contribute to his community in meaningful ways. The role and clinical reasoning of the occupational therapist in supporting Jesse, his family, high school staff, and the employer is described by the occupational therapist. Although this scenario is about one individual with Down syndrome, it is relevant and applicable to many different situations involving youth with different types of disability.

Jesse's Story, Told by His Mother, Jan

Although Jesse was born with a developmental disability, Down syndrome, and is a young man who uses sign language to communicate, he has always been included in the regular classroom at school and taken part in many community organizations in the town where he lives. As his mother, I have been involved with teachers and other professionals who provide support, plan, and strategize ways to make Jesse's participation meaningful to him and an asset to those with whom he learns and works.

After he made a successful transition into high school, we wanted to plan for the day he would graduate. We were concerned that two important outcomes be in place by that time: (1) there would be a mechanism for Jesse that would stimulate friendships and nurture relationships, and (2) he would be involved in meaningful activities where he could contribute to the community.

The vision shared by Jesse and our family is for him to be as independent as possible, have friends, participate in the life of our community, have meaningful activities, such as paid and volunteer work and leisure interests, be valued for who he is, and have a sense of belonging. "Work"

Stewart, D. (Ed.)
*Transitions to Adulthood for Youth With Disabilities
Through an Occupational Therapy Lens (pp. 67-76).*
© 2013 SLACK Incorporated

means much more than paid employment and, in our view, is just one part of a healthy, balanced life. It is important to be able to work, and it is a place where one makes a contribution and is welcomed. Volunteer work is equally important and valued and leads to satisfaction with ourselves and an opportunity to work with others. These aspects of work should be a part of a well-planned, meaningful week for all of us.

Once Jesse entered high school, we began looking for a part-time job similar to the jobs other teenagers were doing at this time in their lives. We received a town newspaper every Sunday and Wednesday delivered by a young adult, and we asked Jesse if this would be something he would be interested in doing. We explained that he would deliver the paper twice a week, that my husband and I would help him, and he would be paid to do so. Jesse thought this was a great idea;we made an appointment to speak to the owner of the newspaper and brought Jesse to his office for an interview. The owner was very welcoming, especially when we told the owner one of us would be with Jesse to support him on the job.

This was Jesse's first paid employment, and it was a great success. He stayed in that job until the paper route ended. Jesse was meticulous in his work and soon began to make friends on his route. In the hot months, neighbors would wait to offer him a cool drink and sometimes he would get a tip. We would stay at the curb while Jesse put the paper in the mailbox or in the homeowner's hand. Jesse made many new acquaintances, provided a service, and was appreciated for his work.

When Jesse was 16 years old, he became eligible for the work experience program at high school. A job coach would be assigned to find placements in different businesses to help Jesse develop his work skills and discover the type of work he would like to do after graduation. At this time we reached out to his former occupational therapist from elementary school who had identified areas in which Jesse needed support in the classroom.

Also at this time, we enrolled Jesse in a workshop called Future Directions presented by the Hamilton Family Network, our parent-to-parent support group. The group offered expertise on how to set up a network for Jesse that would be in place by the time he finished school.. The workshop was held over 4 nights and involved independent planning for Jesse regarding his future. Through the workshop, we learned about various government programs he could apply to for additional support. We were encouraged to invite people close to Jesse, who knew him in different ways from us, to help with the planning. Together, Jesse was able to tell us the types of activities he preferred and the ones he did not like. He was able to tell us the areas where he would need support. For example, he wanted to drive a car. We knew this wasn't possible but one of Jesse's friends, his former swim instructor, suggested Jesse go with him to his grandfather's farm where he could learn to drive their all-terrain vehicle. This made Jesse very happy and was the result of having many people involved in the planning. My husband and I knew we would never have thought of that solution on our own. We brought the ideas garnered from the workshop to our school meetings. Jesse's future began to look interesting, inclusive, and possible.

We had witnessed how lonely life could be for youth with developmental disabilities once they left high school. Suddenly the structure and activity ended, and worse, their friends were dispersed to post-secondary education or employment. We were aware of the success other families had experienced with a structure called Networks of Support, also known as Circle of Friends. This network provided a way to bolster friendships and build relationships.

We invited some of Jesse's good friends from school and the community, as well as friends of our family, to come together to learn what a network is and to consider being a part of one for Jesse. These are the people who know him well and wish to advocate, look out for, and include him in their own lives. The network would come together four times a year, but members would invite Jesse to activities, such as going to the movies, going for a walk, meeting for lunch, or seeing a ball game between meetings. The network provides a social life for Jesse and a "brain-trust" for his parents. For the first time our family had other committed people involved with, and supporting, the many decisions that come along in the life of a person with a disability. Jesse always remains the focus and is encouraged to express his desires and opinions. This was in place by graduation and made the transition out of school much less painful for Jesse.

Through an Occupational Therapy Lens

The Evidence

The literature about youth with developmental disabilities indicates that they are not getting the same opportunities as other youth to participate in productive activities and contribute to their communities (Carey, 2009; Race, 2007). Contributing to one's community in the form of paid or unpaid work is considered by many to be an important aspect of citizenship. Johnson and Walmsley (2010) point out that work is the ultimate badge of citizenship, and people with intellectual disabilities want the opportunity to participate. Recent evidence indicates that employment experiences during high school contribute to improved adult employment opportunities (Hutchinson et al., 2011).

The path to employment and community participation starts in high school, when typically developing students assume volunteer activities and summer jobs. Work-based education (WBE) programs in high schools have evolved over the years to include a number of different options. A recent study of successful WBE programs for youth with developmental disabilities identified four themes:

1. Goals that focus on more than just work.

2. A developmental approach that is proactive and flexible.

3. A focus on building self-advocacy skills for the students.

4. Following best practice guidelines for any work program, such as individualized plans and clear report writing (Hutchinson et al., 2011).

Adolescents with intellectual disabilities face numerous environmental challenges that limit their employment experiences (Burbridge, Minnes, Buell, & Ouellette-Kuntz, 2008). Volunteer activities can provide an alternative option for productive community activity. From an occupational therapy perspective, productive occupations of any kind (paid or unpaid) provide key elements of citizenship, such as self-determination, participation, and contribution (Kirsch et al., 2009) (Figure 4-1). Therefore, it is important to find the best match for each student to optimize his or her participation in the workplace and community at large.

The Occupational Therapist's View of Occupation, Spirituality, and Development for Jesse

Jesse was a student whom I knew for a number of years through my work as an occupational therapist in the elementary and secondary school system, prior to this work experience placement. Now the school and family were preparing Jesse for a life of active community participation when he graduated. Everyone wanted Jesse to have a "meaningful" week, where he could be fully involved and contributing as a community member. Jesse was at a developmental stage of readiness for this transition.

The journey toward adulthood typically involves occupations related to work. In high school, there are often options for students who are preparing for future work, such as *co-op placements*, which are counted as credit courses. In our local school board, there is a *work experience* program, with some similarities to co-op, provided for students with disabilities to support their transition to the adult world. Whatever challenges his or her disability presents, no student is seen as unsuitable for a work experience placement. This type of positive and strengths-based attitude is

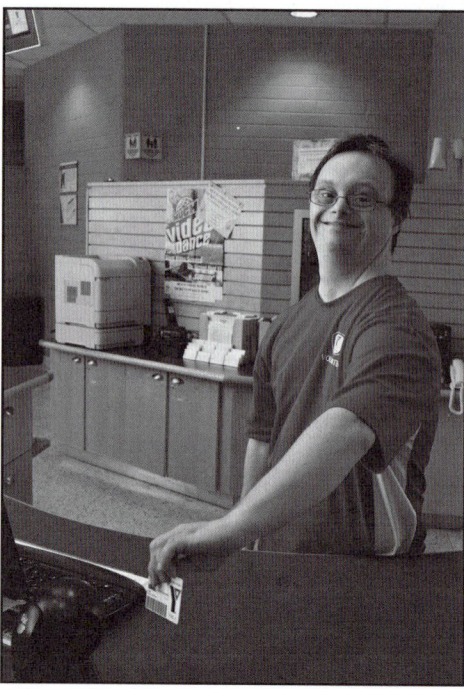

Figure 4-1. Contributing to the community through work is an important aspect of citizenship.

important, because educators and other professionals who judge that certain individuals "won't benefit" from a community placement can be the main barriers to a successful transition for youth with developmental disabilities. Their attitudes often reflect their own skepticism about inclusion for everyone.

This work experience program has had unprecedented success over the years in promoting integration for the most challenged students and in showing the community it can be done. Young adults, who previously left school with a bleak future, can now graduate with a vision and a viable plan for community participation, volunteering, and work. The work experience program is led by a transition coordinator, who works with all the high schools around their planning for special needs students. The coordinator sources the placements, supervises the team of job coaches, matches the students with the placement, and liaises with parents and the school.

Person-Environment-Occupation Analysis

Prior to a student beginning a work experience, there are meetings at the school. Members of the transition planning team knew Jesse in different ways—as a student, a friend, an assistant, a son, etc.—so they would all have different contributions to make. My input was related to Jesse's abilities and support needs in the context of various work settings. However, we could all talk about his personality and interests, and the pros and cons of different placements. Jesse, of course, participated in meetings, as we all endorse the "People First" motto: "Nothing About Me Without Me" (Institute on Human Development and Disability, n.d.). The grocery store closest to Jesse's home was chosen for his placement. The transition coordinator met with the manager to discuss which area of the store could best accommodate him. The produce department was selected. This was a good location for Jesse for several reasons. It was a spacious area on the perimeter of the store, with room to move about and for the job coach and Jesse to work side by side. Jesse was in a place with high visibility and good possibilities for customer and staff interactions.

My role at this stage was to provide an occupational profile (American Occupational Therapy Association [AOTA], 2008) of Jesse, which offered a summary of information about his occupational performance. This included his occupational experiences, history, patterns, interests, values, and needs (AOTA, 2008). I used a person-environment-occupation (PEO) analysis framework to document information about Jesse in a report that was useful and easily understood by the school staff and store manager. The following information was included.

Person

Jesse was 17 years old at the time of this placement, living at home with his parents and younger sister. Jesse's mother, Jan, told me about his current performance patterns. He was attending an inclusive high school in his community. In addition to regular classes, Jesse participated in the drama club and loved to go to school football games and dances with his friends. He was a happy student with a strong sense of belonging and contribution to school life.

Jesse was able to perform his own personal hygiene but needed help shaving and shampooing. He ate a well-rounded but soft diet and fed himself. Jesse enjoyed swimming, hiking, bowling, and canoeing in the summer. He worked out at the YMCA on the fitness machines and did some weightlifting. He loved walking and had a great long-distance walking tolerance.

I also gathered current information about Jesse's performance skills and personal factors. My observations of Jesse in different situations indicated that his motor skills were adequate for most daily activities. Jesse had low muscle tone overall, but with exercise, he was able to maintain good muscle strength and range of motion in all extremities. He did experience some difficulties with praxis skills, as his hand-eye coordination and manipulation skills were slow. He usually required supervision to follow through on complex verbal commands or to complete a temporal sequence of activities.

Jesse has Down syndrome, which influences cognitive skills such as judging, organizing, remembering, and multitasking. In most cases, he needed personal assistance to complete tasks that involved complex cognitive functions.

Jesse was able to express himself through sign language and nonverbal communication. His parents reported that he had a positive outlook on life and enjoyed interacting with peers and family members. He was shy in new social situations, but over time he gained confidence and began to communicate with people in new environments.

It was important in this initial report to highlight the personal strengths and assets that Jesse was bringing to this situation, but also to identify the performance areas in which he would need support and/or adaptations.

Environment

For this situation, it was important to consider the physical, social, and cultural aspects of the environment.

In the grocery store setting, some physical considerations were as follows:

- Mode of transportation to and from the placement
- Impact of inclement weather
- The entrance door—weight and manual versus automatic opening
- The sign-in procedure and location of sign-in book
- Staff room layout (i.e., cupboards and refrigerator)
- Physical features and overall layout (i.e., noise levels, location of loading area for produce and cardboard recycle, etc.)

Several social and cultural features of the workplace had to be considered. I observed the workplace environment to identify opportunities for the job coach to support Jesse in interactions with customers and staff. At the beginning, the family and occupational therapist felt it was best for Jesse and the job coach to make their way into work quietly and unobtrusively. It was not necessary to talk further with the manager or to put anything else in place. Students with disabilities can often advocate for themselves through their own contributions when we give them opportunities in the right setting. Once Jesse had been working for awhile and everyone noticed how smoothly things were going, the opportunity was there to ask the manager about Jesse continuing to work when school was finished.

Occupation

Jesse was travelling by bus from the school with his job coach and crossing a busy street to enter the store. We were pleased to see that Jesse had already learned to sign in and go upstairs to the staff room to put on his shirt and name tag. The job coach had requested that Jesse follow the same procedures as others and wear his name tag to identify his status as a worker.

There were many different jobs to be done in the produce department, some more complex than others. Some jobs required lifting and moving, many required skill in the use of a knife (trimming), and others demanded experience and judgment (e.g., layout and display placement). The produce manager suggested that putting out potatoes would be an appropriate task to begin with, so this was where Jesse started.

An occupational analysis focuses on the specific occupations that a person wants to or needs to perform in different environments. This level of analysis includes social roles and the meaning of the occupation for the person, as this will greatly influence his or her performance (Crepeau, Cohn, & Boyt Schell, 2009; Watson & Wilson, 2003). For Jesse and his family, the meaning of this work experience went far beyond the development of job skills, focusing on relationships, participation, and contributions to the community. This opportunity was providing valuable experience for future adult roles as a worker, and just as importantly, as a community member and citizen.

At the level of task analysis, I reviewed the main steps and sequence for each job, including putting out potatoes (Figure 4-2). The first step was moving the potatoes already out on the table to the front (rotation). Next the trolley was taken to the back of the store to load several boxes of fresh potatoes. These were added to the display table in a visually pleasing manner (i.e., evenly distributed and not spilling into other produce). The usual process was to dump out the boxes, but Jesse used a slower and more deliberate method of placing them by hand. After this, the boxes were taken to the back of the store, flattened, and stacked for bundling and recycling.

Theoretical Approaches

Based on this PEO analysis, there were three theoretical approaches that would be appropriate for this situation. A cognitive-neurological approach would address the challenges in finding the best fit between Jesse's cognitive abilities and the cognitive demands of the occupation. A sociocultural approach would address the issues related to the fit between the social aspects of the environment, the social demands of being a grocery clerk, and Jesse's current social skills. An environmental approach would be needed at times to address the needs of the store staff and customers who were not used to having a young person with a disability, and a job coach, in his or her environment.

All of these theoretical approaches could be used at different times, and together sometimes, to ensure that the next stages of assessment and intervention covered all aspects of Jesse's work experience. The three theoretical approaches (cognitive-neurological, sociocultural, and environmental) led to ongoing task/activity analysis, clinical observations, discussions with team members, and different task and environmental modifications. No "fine tuning" was necessary along the way, as these three approaches were appropriate for assessment and intervention.

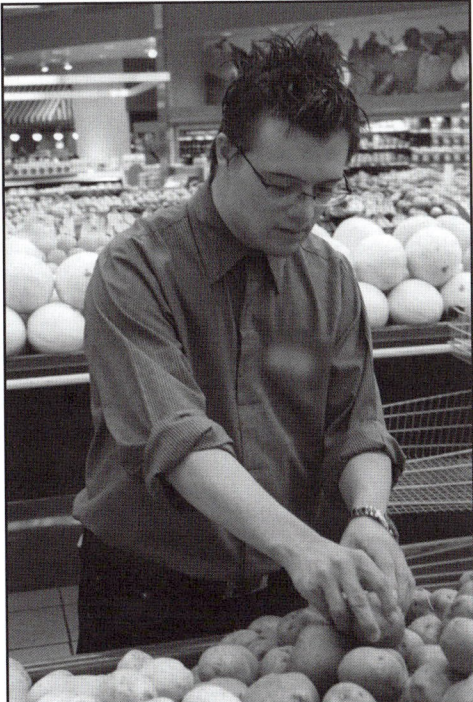

Figure 4-2. Work in a produce department involves numerous tasks.

Assessment and Intervention

A dynamic approach to assessment and intervention fit best with the complex and interactional elements of this situation. This approach is challenging for the therapist, but is also highly flexible and adaptable for the people we are working with. A dynamic assessment process works well in times of transition, as it encourages a flexible individualized process that focuses on learning and change (Toglia, Golisz, & Goverover, 2009). The occupational therapist "uses cues, mediation, feedback, or alterations of activity demands" (Toglia et al., 2009, p. 743) to determine an individual's full range of performance potential. The therapist would change one element (within the PEO) of the person's performance at a time. If this change makes a positive difference, then the therapist can employ cueing or mediation strategies to improve the person's performance over time. This illustrates how dynamic assessment results can interact with and inform intervention (Toglia et al., 2009).

The focus of intervention was not primarily on the development of job skills but on enabling Jesse's participation and contribution in a work setting, in order to help prepare him for a satisfying adult life. The intervention approach was consultative. Those in the school system who were in day-to-day contact with Jesse would be "direct service" providers—the teachers, job coach, educational assistants, and so on. Typically the occupational therapist would have limited direct involvement with the student, but would offer expertise in the form of strategies, suggestions, detailed task analysis, and a breakdown of steps to promote new learning.

Consultation is considered to be a key enablement skill (Townsend, Beagan, & Kumas-Tau, 2007), and it involves an exchange of views and ideas with a range of people. It fits well with an environmental approach, as strategies may involve adapting the environment or tasks to improve a student's performance (Bazyk & Case-Smith, 2010). The following is an example of how this service approach was implemented.

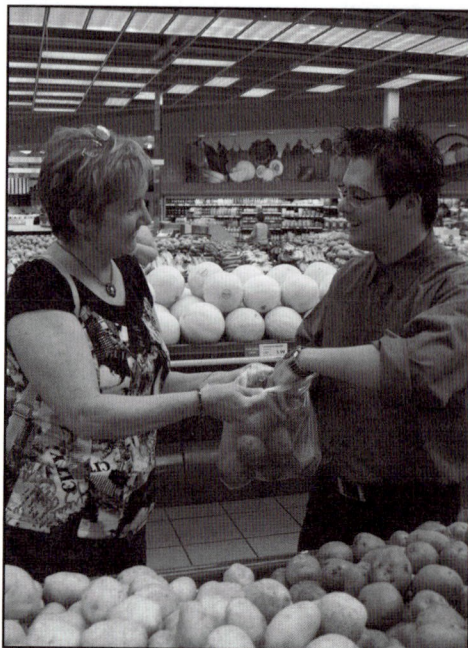

Figure 4-3. Interactions with customers are part of the work experience in a grocery store setting.

I noticed that customers often hesitated to approach and speak with Jesse, thinking they might be interrupting instruction from the job coach. Additionally, staff tended to address the job coach rather than Jesse directly. I believed that Jesse could use some support in developing working relations with store staff and customers. I worked with the job coach to make this happen (Figure 4-3). The job coach tried to support rather than impede Jesse's interactions with customers and staff. The job coach's role was to facilitate opportunities for Jesse to build this bridge himself, which Jesse did by his quiet presence and warm smile. I also spent some of my time sitting with Jesse and staff at break times, as this offered an opportunity to speak together and get past mutual shyness.

Conclusion

Jesse was working. He was being challenged to learn new skills, to become more independent, and to experience what life would be like after school. However, he was at this grocery store for a more important reason than work. He was there to find his place in the "community" of people surrounding him; to experience the relationships and connections, the social opportunities and requirements, and everything involved in "belonging" to a culture of work. In return, he would benefit from the acceptance and respect of others, the camaraderie, and the satisfaction of making a contribution. This work experience led to a part-time job after he graduated from high school, which was a positive outcome. Of equal importance, Jesse now belonged to a community. He was invited to staff social events and was well known to the customers, who were members of his larger community.

Measuring outcomes in this dynamic systems approach meant that a formal outcome measure was not necessary. Rather, the occupational therapist gathered outcome information as part of the ongoing process of assessment and treatment. Qualitative methods, such as interviews and observations, were used to learn about the experiences and perceptions of Jesse, his job coach, the transition coordinator, store manager, and family members. This information was then organized

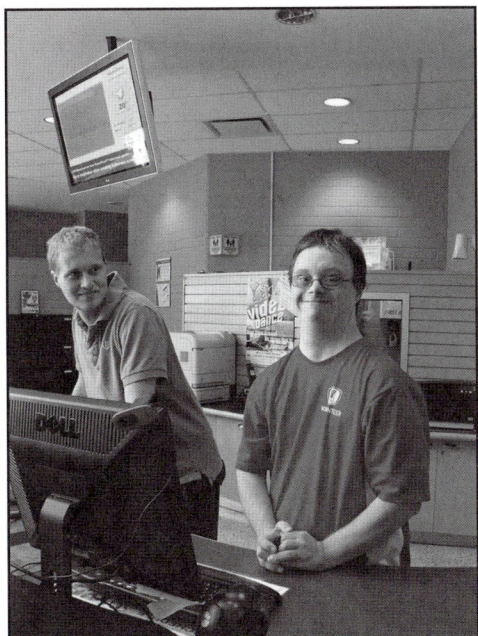

Figure 4-4. Jesse and his job coach at the YMCA.

into outcome "themes" of participation, contributions, relationships, and belonging for Jesse. This also included outcomes for the community, such as other people's capacity to include Jesse in regular workplace activities.

In conclusion, a dynamic approach to occupational therapy assessment and intervention was effective in helping Jesse achieve his goal of contributing to his community through a meaningful work experience. This type of approach could also be used to address other aspects of Jesse's adult life. For example, when Jesse wanted to get exercise after graduating from high school, he went to the YMCA to go swimming and to work out regularly. Through observation, interviews, and task analysis, an occupational therapist could assist in helping Jesse to participate and contribute in this setting (Figure 4-4).

Jan's Description of Outcomes for Jesse Summarizes This Best

With the thoughtful, step-by-step preparation of the occupational therapist, Jesse was able to have a successful work experience at the grocery store. It was so successful that he was invited to stay on after high school graduation. He was also able to transfer some of the skills he learned to other workplace and community opportunities. After he had been at the YMCA for a while, the manager invited Jesse to be a host at the reception desk, as his smile and pleasant nature welcomed everyone as he swiped his or her membership card.

Jesse was a person who was easily overwhelmed by complicated tasks and strangers, but after being on the job for a few months he developed confidence and began seeing himself as an adult worker. His demeanor before this work experience was keeping his head down and his eyes on the floor. His new self-confidence brought his gaze up to meet other people's eyes, which was wonderful for our family to see.

Jesse changed from a shy, passive individual to a smiling, confident young man who was happy to go to work and do his job. Working at the grocery store brought Jesse into contact with shoppers who started to greet him and smile to let him know they appreciated what he was doing. Jesse's sense of belonging and feeling valued for his contribution greatly eased his transition into the adult world. As for us, his family, it was great to see him participating happily and taking his place in our community.

Review Questions

1. What did work mean to Jesse and his family? What was work's role and significance in his life?

2. How does the occupational therapist view work and its impact on Jesse's overall well-being?

3. Describe a work-based experience program in high schools. Who is involved? What is the process? Is it successful?

4. What was the occupational therapist's role in the work-based experience program?

5. What assessments and interventions did the occupational therapist use and why?

References

American Occupational Therapy Association (AOTA). (2008). *Occupational therapy practice framework: Domain and process* (2nd ed.). Bethesda, MD: American Occupational Therapy Association Press.

Bazyk, S., & Case-Smith, J. (2010). School-based occupational therapy. In J. Case-Smith & J. C. O'Brien (Eds.), *Occupational therapy for children* (6th ed., pp. 713-742). St. Louis, MO: Elsevier.

Burbridge, J., Minnes, P., Buell, K., & Ouellette-Kuntz, H. (2008). Preparing to leave school: Involvement of students with intellectual disabilities in productive activities. *Journal on Developmental Disabilities, 14*(1), 19-26.

Carey, A. C. (2009). *On the margins of citizenship: Intellectual disability and civil rights in twentieth-century America.* Philadelphia, PA: Temple University Press.

Crepeau, E. B., Cohn, E. S., & Boyt Schell, B. A. (Eds.). (2009). *Willard and Spackman's occupational therapy* (11th ed.). New York, NY: Lippincott Williams & Wilkins.

Hutchinson, N. L., Versnel, J., Poth, C., Berg, D., deLugta, J., Daltona, C. J., Chin, P., & Munby, H. (2011). They want to come to school: Work-based education programs to prevent the social exclusion of vulnerable youth. *Work, 40*(2), 195-209.

Institute on Human Development and Disability. (n.d.). *Nothing about me without me.* Retrieved from www.ihdd.uga.edu/DisabilityRightsAdvocacy/DRAHome.html

Johnson, K., & Walmsley, J. (2010). *People with intellectual disabilities: Towards a good life?* Portland, OR: Policy Press.

Kirsh, B., Stergiou-Kita, M., Gewurtz, R., Dawson, D., Krupa, T., Lysaght, R., & Shaw, L. (2009). From margins to mainstream: What do we know about work integration for persons with brain injury, mental illness and intellectual disability? *Work, 32*(4), 391-405. doi: 10.3233/WOR-2009-0851

Race, D. (2007). *Intellectual disability: Social approaches.* Maidenhead, UK: McGraw-Hill.

Toglia, J. P., Golisz, K. M., & Goverover, Y. (2009). Evaluation and intervention for cognitive perceptual impairments. In E. B. Crepeau, E. S. Cohn, & B. A. Boyt Schell (Eds.), *Willard and Spackman's occupational therapy* (11th ed., pp. 739-776). New York, NY: Lippincott Williams & Wilkins.

Townsend, E. A., Beagan, B., Kumas-Tan, Z., Versnel, J., Iwama, M., Landry, J.,...Brown, J. (2007). Enabling: Occupational therapy's core competency. In E. A. Townsend & H. J. Polatajko (Eds.), *Enabling occupation II: Advancing an occupational therapy vision for health, well-being, and justice through occupation* (pp. 87-133). Ottawa, Ontario, Canada: CAOT Publications ACE.

Watson, D. E., & Wilson, S. (2003). *Task analysis: An individual and population approach* (2nd ed.). Bethesda, MD: American Occupational Therapy Association Press.

Transition to Post-Secondary Education for Youth With Learning Disabilities Using Assistive Technology

Baljit Samrai, MSc, BSc, BHSc, OT Reg (Ont);
Kim Carey, Hons B Kin, OT Reg (Ont); and Christy Taberner, OT Reg (Ont)

The purpose of this chapter is to demonstrate how occupational therapists are ideally suited to work with youth who have learning disabilities. When working with students, occupational therapists are able to use their unique occupational therapy lens of person-environment-occupation (PEO) to make recommendations for optimal participation and inclusion in the school environment. In addition, occupational therapists can play an integral role in helping clients understand their personal strengths and challenges for academic learning. This awareness is essential in order to help individuals advocate for their learning needs as they transition from high school to the post-secondary environment.

The scenario in this chapter is about an occupational therapist working in a school health services program who has received a referral for Jessica, a 17-year-old girl with a diagnosis of attention deficit disorder (ADD) with a coexisting diagnosis of a learning disability. The referral was sent by the school board following a meeting with Jessica's parents, who requested support for Jessica's successful completion of high school and preparation for post-secondary education. The occupational therapist has a total of four visits to assess Jessica's needs and make recommendations. Afterward, further sessions for the implementation of recommendations would be determined.

Introducing Jessica

Hi, my name is Jessica, and I am 17 years old. I've always strived to be the best that I can. I have received lots of help at home and at school. Sometimes the help I need is to have someone explain something when I just don't understand what I have read. So, I have had some problems with homework, creating projects, trying to remember things, and sometimes I feel I get lost in all the

Stewart, D. (Ed.)
Transitions to Adulthood for Youth With Disabilities
Through an Occupational Therapy Lens (pp. 77-102).

details. At home, my mom and older siblings help me. My mom was very patient with me when she helped with my homework; whereas my siblings would just do it for me instead of helping me. At school, I've had some support from an educational assistant, and she was great at helping me come up with ideas, pointing out things I had missed, and keeping me on track. I have a few close friends at high school, and for the most part I enjoy going to school. My parents think I should go to college after high school, and my friends have talked about continuing with their education too; I think I will plan to do the same. I haven't quite figured out what I will study, although I have always thought I'd like to be a paramedic. I am concerned about how am I going to manage at college.

Occupation, Spirituality, and Development

It is through the everyday process of engaging in roles that adolescents develop both independence and interdependence (Vroman, 2010). One of the primary occupations of an adolescent is that of a student. Engagement in this role contributes to developmental tasks of independence and interdependence. As students, adolescents test their skills and abilities as they learn about themselves and identify which academic areas interest them and in which areas they have proficiency. This process eventually leads to narrowing their interests in regards to occupational choices. As school becomes increasingly challenging, they are required to take greater responsibility for studying and performing academically. They are expected to function more independently with each year of progression (middle and secondary grades). If they choose to go on to post-secondary education, the demands for them to be more responsible for their own learning are greater. The student role also provides adolescents with opportunities to develop interdependence as they work collaboratively with other students to accomplish group projects and to work in study groups.

Participation in school-related occupations can provide adolescents with opportunities to engage in roles other than that of a student. Related roles that can occur within the context of a school environment include friend, club or organization member, leader, teammate, and boyfriend or girlfriend. These roles involve significant occupation and task demands that contribute to the development of identity, capacities and talents, leadership skills, and vocational interests. The emerging concept of occupational development acknowledges that the *dynamics of doing* that is part of occupational performance can influence an individual's abilities in context (Humphry, 2009).

Higher education is viewed as a critical stepping stone by which people can improve their status in life. Furthermore, post-secondary credentials may be indicators of future potential (Levine & Nourse, 1998). When students are making the transition from high school to post-secondary education, they will experience significant changes in the occupations that bring meaning and purpose to their lives. A person's goal of attaining further education at a post-secondary level can have a multitude of meanings such as the following:

» Developing a sense of accomplishment and success

» Benefitting from experiential learning, for lifelong learning

» Promoting skills in problem solving, decision making, and personal management for all facets of adult life

» Development of self-advocacy skills

» Increasing a sense of self-awareness, self-worth, and identity

» Development of adult social skills

For youth with disabilities, there may be some additional meanings associated with post-secondary education, such as exercising their right to participate in a socially inclusive environment (Townsend & Polatajko, 2007), and learning to identify and deal with environmental barriers that can limit full participation. Research about the post-high school outcomes of youth with learning disabilities has found that these youth are at a disadvantage, compared to youth without disabilities, and often do not achieve their aspirations of post-secondary education (Learning Disabilities Association of Canada [LDAC], 2007; Wagner, Newman, Cameto, Levine, & Garza, 2006). The rate of post-secondary enrollment for youth with learning disabilities has increased in the past decade or so, but it is still significantly less than their peers (Riddell, Tinklin & Wilson, 2005; Wagner et al., 2006). Youth who do enter into post-secondary education may find a mix of supports and barriers to full participation (Riddell et al., 2005). For example, Killean and Hubka (1999) surveyed post-secondary students with disabilities from across Canada and found that the majority were receiving some form of academic accommodations. The participants identified academic support services and adaptive technology as supports, and the lack of a disability services office as a barrier (Killean & Hubka, 1999).

How Does a Learning Disability Affect the Student Role?

Definition of a Learning Disability

It is estimated that learning disabilities affect 5% to 10% of Canadians and Americans (LDAC, 2007; Rogers, 2010). *Learning disability* is defined by the National Joint Committee on Learning Disabilities (1990 p. 3) as,

> *A general term that refers to a heterogeneous group of disorders manifested by significant difficulties in the acquisition and use of listening, speaking, reading, writing, reasoning, or mathematical abilities. These disorders are intrinsic to the individual, presumed to be due to central nervous system dysfunction, and may occur across the life span. Problems in self-regulatory behaviors, social perception, and social interaction may exist with learning disabilities but do not by themselves constitute a learning disability. Although learning disabilities may occur concomitantly with other handicapping conditions (for example, sensory impairment, mental retardation, serious emotional disturbance), or with extrinsic influences (such as cultural differences, insufficient or inappropriate instruction), they are not the result of those conditions or influences.*

Learning disabilities range in severity and invariably interfere with many activities of daily living (ADL). One area, in which the effects of a learning disability are especially prominent, is in the area of academic performance. Current evidence (Shapiro, Church, & Lewis, 2007) indicates that the primary psychological processes that impact learning include the following:

» Phonological/language processing: The ability to identify and manipulate sounds into words, including language reception, expression, oral, and written.

» Memory and attention: The ability to attend to, store, hold, and recall/retrieve information. This includes visual, auditory, phonological, working, and short- and long-term memory.

» Processing speed: Speed of intake of information and understanding, using, or responding to information. The ability to perform simple cognitive or perceptual tasks rapidly and efficiently. This measures how efficiently one learns.

» Visual-spatial processing: The ability to process visual stimuli and to analyze, discriminate, and interpret visual patterns and designs.

» Perceptual-motor processing: The ability to use sensory feedback to guide physical movements.

» Executive functions: The ability to plan, organize, efficiently manage time, and evaluate one's progress and performance (i.e., problem solving).

Impairments in these areas invariably interfere with the acquisition and use of one or more of the following important academic-related skills:

> » Oral language (listening, speaking, understanding)

> » Reading (decoding, comprehension)

> » Written language (spelling, written expression)

> » Mathematics (computation, problem solving)

> » Organization (planning, initiation, completion of task, time management)

An individual's ability to participate in ADL requires the integration of these important skills. Consequently, difficulty in these aforementioned psychological processes will impact an individual's ability to participate in many of his or her everyday occupations. Learning disabilities vary greatly in terms of impairment and impact on academic, social, and emotional functioning.

How Is a Learning Disability Diagnosed?

Impairments caused by learning disabilities are usually present for life. However, the impact of the disability may be seen at different times across the lifespan, depending on the environmental and occupational demands placed upon an individual. Some impairment's may be observed during early school years; others may emerge at a later time in an individual's academic career. Often learning disabilities are first suspected when there is an unexpectedly low academic achievement or achievement that is only sustainable with extreme effort and support (Learning Disabilities Association of Ontario [LDAO], 2011).

Once a learning disability is suspected, an individual may be referred for psychoeducational testing by a registered psychologist or designated psychological associate in order to obtain a diagnosis (LDAO, 2011). A thorough psychoeducational assessment is critical to identify a person's unique learning strengths and challenges as well as to obtain recommendations with respect to enhancing learning that are unique to that person's profile.

Assistive Technology

The use of assistive technology (AT) is a compensatory strategy that is used in all education systems to support the needs of students who have learning disabilities. Evidence supports the use of AT, along with academic accommodations and support services, as the most successful strategies in supporting the needs of these students (Batorowicz, Missiuna, & Pollock, accepted; Killean & Hubka, 1999).

In the United States, AT is legally defined in Public Law 108-364 (The Assistive Technology Act of 1998, amended) as "any item, piece of equipment, or product system, whether acquired commercially or off the shelf modified or customized, that is used to increase or improve functional capabilities of individuals with disabilities" (Schoonover, Argabrite, Grove, & Swinth, 2010, p. 584). Some devices compensate for a functional deficit, such as an alternative communication device for persons without speech, or a wheelchair to mobilize independently if someone cannot walk. Cognitive prostheses are a form of technology that replaces or circumvents an ability that is absent or impaired. For example, audio feedback on the computer can help a student with a reading disability to translate text into meaningful information, and voice recognition can assist a student who cannot input text through a keyboard. The use of AT in these situations can facilitate the student's move toward independence by reducing his or her reliance on others to perform tasks such as reading, writing, listening, and organizing (Mull & Sitlington, 2003).

Computers are often prescribed as an alternative to handwriting, and occupational therapists are often part of the interdisciplinary team involved in the evaluation and prescription of these devices (Schoonover et al., 2010). Handwriting is a very complex task that requires the student to integrate postural control with visual and motor abilities. These physical demands combined with the attention, memory, and other cognitive and language demands are often overwhelming for students with learning difficulties. A student who experiences difficulty with this task may experience decreased feelings of confidence and lowered self-esteem as a result of performing below the levels of his or her peers (McHale & Cermak, 1992 as cited in Chwirka, Gurney, & Brutner, 2002), which could ultimately impact academic performance. Keyboarding and the use of computers are even more important for children who have a combination of coordination and learning difficulties.

Person-Environment-Occupation Analysis and Theoretical Approaches

Prior to the initial interview with Jessica, the occupational therapist reviews the following relevant documentation provided with Jessica's file to gather information about her occupational performance and specific performance components in the academic setting:

1. Psychoeducational assessment report (review and interpret results)

2. Current Individualized Education Plan (IEP)

3. Consultation notes from Jessica's current learning resource teacher

The occupational therapist also interviews Jessica and her parents in order to obtain the following information:

1. Perspectives on academic performance and school functioning in relation to her occupational performance, through administration of the Canadian Occupational Performance Measure (COPM) (Law, 2005). Other measures of occupational performance could also be used at this stage.

2. Interpretation of the key results of the psychoeducational assessment findings and what this means for Jessica's academic functioning.

3. Identification of Jessica's strengths and weaknesses and environmental supports and barriers via administration of the COPM.

The results from these two methods of data collection and assessment provide the occupational therapist with a great deal of information that requires synthesis and interpretation for the therapist, Jessica, and her family.

Summary of Psychoeducational Results

The occupational therapist reviews the findings from the psychoeducational report and then organizes them into a visual bell curve (Figure 5-1). This visual representation of the psychoeducational results serves to summarize the key findings of this assessment and to present them in a way that is easier to understand than the raw data (Table 5-1).

During the initial visit with the client, it is beneficial for the occupational therapist to review the results of the psychoeducational report with the family. Often, the youth and his or her parents do not fully understand the findings in the report, and an occupational therapist can often help in translating the findings into functional implications. This is the case for Jessica and her parents. In the first visit, she said that she did not really understand what the report meant for her, other than getting extra help at school.

Functional Implications of Psychoeducational Assessment

Overall, the findings indicate that Jessica has age-appropriate reasoning skills, but is experiencing difficulty with being an efficient learner due to slow processing speed and poor working and

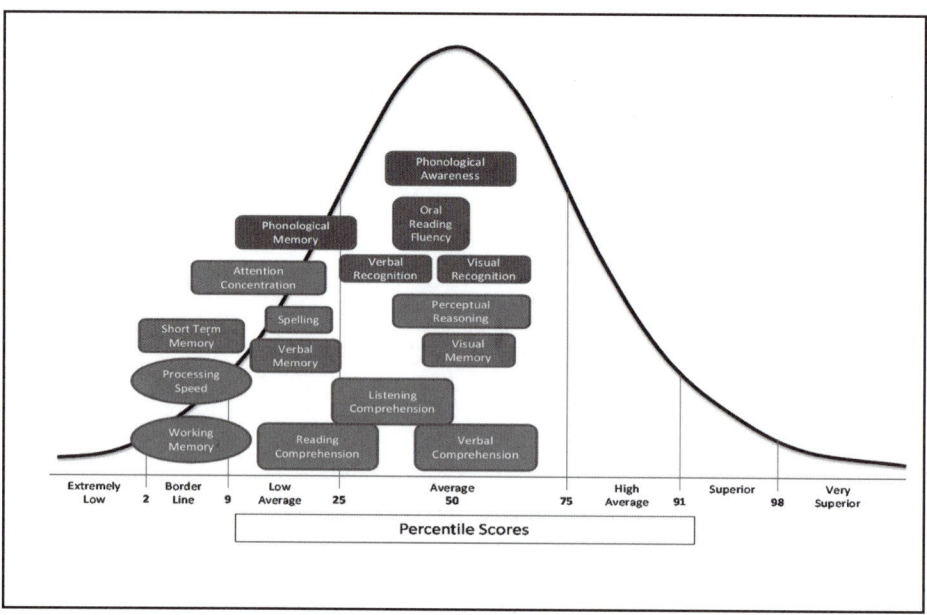

Figure 5-1. Graphic presentation of Jessica's performance of key areas of the psychoeducational assessment.

Table 5-1.			
Psychoeducational Assessment Results			
Test Administered	**Description**	**Percentile Rank**	**Category**
Wechsler Adult Intelligence Scales, 4th edition (WAIS-IV)	Tests overall cognitive/intellectual skills using 15 subtests.	21	Low average
	Verbal comprehension (measuring language based skills)	50	Average
	Vocabulary—Give verbal definition of words measuring expressive vocabulary skills	63	Average
	Similarities—Measures verbal conceptual reasoning skills by indicating how various concepts are similar	50	Average
	Information—Questions presented orally measuring one's overall general knowledge	37	Average
	Comprehension—Questions are presented orally to assess social judgment and understanding of cause and effect relationships	N/A	

(continued)

Table 5-1 (continued).			
Psychoeducational Assessment Results			
Test Administered	**Description**	**Percentile Rank**	**Category**
Wechsler Adult Intelligence Scales, 4th edition (WAIS-IV)	Perceptual reasoning (measuring visually mediated skills)	23	Below average
	1. Block design—Measures visual/spatial reasoning skills by making designs with blocks that are visually presented on a series of cards	12	Below average
	2. Matrix reasoning—Measures visual spatial perception and fluid reasoning by the individual examining an incomplete matrix design and choosing the one (from an array of 5) that best completes the design	23	Below average
	3. Visual puzzles—Measures visual spatial skills by presenting a diagram and then having the individual determine which 3 pictures go together to make the diagram	34	Average
	4. Figure weights—Measures fluid reasoning by having the individual view a scale to determine which option keeps the scale balanced	N/A	
	5. Picture completion—Assesses attention to visual detail by having the individual indicate the missing elements of familiar pictures	N/A	
	Working memory subtest (measuring the ability to mentally manipulate information within a small time span)	5	Borderline
	1. Digit span—Measures short-term memory by assessing an individual's ability to repeat a series of numbers increasing in length in a forwards and backwards manner as well as recall numbers in an ascending order	9	Below average
	2. Arithmetic—Assesses mental computation skills and short-term memory by completing an oral arithmetic test	9	Below average
	3. Letter number sequencing—Measures auditory working memory by requiring the individual to recall a series of letters and numbers of increasing length and having them reorder the items in a number first then letter fashion, then both must be recalled in a numerical and alphabetical order, respectively	N/A	

(continued)

Table 5-1 (continued).			
Psychoeducational Assessment Results			
Test Administered	**Description**	**Percentile Rank**	**Category**
Wechsler Adult Intelligence Scales, 4th edition (WAIS-IV)	Processing speed subtest (measures speed and accuracy)	8	Borderline
	1. Coding—Measures speed of visual processing by completing a copying task (copy symbols that corresponds to specific numbers (within a time limit)	16	Below average
	2. Symbol search—Measures visual processing speed by completing a pencil and paper scanning test where they have to indicate whether a target stimulus is present in an array of stimuli	9	Below average
	3. Cancellation—The individual has to cross off all the picture of animals that he or she sees amongst other pictures as quickly as possible	N/A	
Wide Range Assessment of Memory & Learning, 2nd edition (WRAML-II)	Assesses memory skills in different areas. Consists of 9 core tests and 4 supplemental tests		
	General memory index is derived from verbal memory index and visual memory index	6	Borderline
	Verbal memory index—Contains 2 subtests	9	Low average
	1. Recall 2 short stories		
	2. Learn a list of words over 4 trials		
	Delayed recall scores = the clients' ability to recall the short stories and word series after a short delay	25	Average
	Visual memory index—Contains 2 subtests	42	Average
	1. Reproduce designs after a 10-second delay	50	Average
	2. Immediately indicate changes in pictures they saw	37	Average
	Attention/concentration index—Required to immediately reproduce a series of visual sequences and rote recall a series of numbers and letters	4	Borderline
	Verbal recognition index—Involves multiple choice and true/false questions presented verbally which measure the ability to recognize details from the 2 stories and word series learned previously (verbal memory index, see above)	37	Average
	Visual recognition index—Involves multiple choice and true/false questions to determine the ability to recognize designs and pictures previously seen (visual memory index, see above)	50	Average
	General recognition index = verbal recognition index + visual recognition index		Average

(continued)

Table 5-1 (continued).			
Psychoeducational Assessment Results			
Test Administered	**Description**	**Percentile Rank**	**Category**
Wechsler Individual Achievement Test–III (WIAT-III)	Made up of 16 subtests measuring listening, reading, writing, and math skills		
	Please note: Scores between 16th and 84th percentile for this test are considered average		
	Listening comprehension—Matching a picture with verbal presented concepts, followed by answering questions about an audio recording of a short passage	4	Average
	Oral expression—Naming concepts in visually presented pictures, then the student says words from a given category and repeats sentences	53	Average
	Reading comprehension—Involves answering open-ended questions after reading a passage	47	Below average
	Word reading—Reads a list of increasingly difficult words aloud	23	Average
	Pseudo-word decoding—Reads a list of increasingly difficult nonsense words aloud	2	Below average
	Oral reading fluency—Answers comprehension questions orally after reading a passage aloud	16	Average
	Sentence composition—Involves writing meaningful sentences using specific words and then combines information from 2 or 3 sentences into a single sentence that means the same thing	53	Average
	Essay composition—Writes an essay within 10 minutes	84	High average
	Spelling—Writes single words that are dictated within the context of a sentence to clarify meaning	8	Below average
	Math problem solving—The student is asked to solve math problems related to basic skills (counting, discriminating shapes, etc.) in everyday application (e.g., time and money), geometry, and algebra without time restriction: the task is presented relative to the individual's grade and ability level .	18	Average
	Numerical operation—Involves solving written math problems in the following areas: basic skills, basic operations with integers, geometry, algebra, and calculus without a time restriction and is presented according to grade and ability.	9	Below average
	Math fluency—Addition, subtraction, and multiplication—Involves solving written addition, subtraction, and multiplication problems within a 60-second time limit	5	Below average

(continued)

	Table 5-1 (continued).		
	Psychoeducational Assessment Results		
Test Administered	**Description**	**Percentile Rank**	**Category**
Comprehensive Test of Phonological Processing (CTOPP)	Test deficits in phonological awareness, memory, and rapid naming		
	Phonological awareness—2 subtests	27	Average
	1. Elison test—The individual is presented with a word and then asked to repeat the word without particular sounds	50	Average
	2. Blending words—The individual is presented with two words and is required to blend them together to sound the target word	16	Low average
	Phonological memory—2 subtests	12	Low average
	1. Memory for digits—Recall a series of numbers with increasing complexity	9	Low average
	2. Nonsense word repetition—Repetition of nonsense words of increasing complexity	25	Average
	Rapid naming—2 subtests	12	Low average
	1. Rapid digit naming—Quickly naming a series of numbers	16	Low average
	2. Rapid letter naming—Quickly naming a series of letters	16	Low average
Delis-Kaplan Executive Function System (DKEFS)	Typically 9 tests measuring verbal and non-verbal executive functions; for the purpose of this assessment only 2 are presented.		
	Verbal fluency test—Has 3 test conditions		
	1. Letter fluency—Individual is asked to generate words that begin with a particular letter as quickly as possible	98	Very superior
	2. Category fluency—Individual is asked to generate words that belong to a designated semantic category as quickly as possible	99	Very superior
	3. Category switching—Individual is asked to generate words alternating between 2 different semantic categories as quickly as possible	63	Average
	The color-word interference test—Has 4 subtests measuring quick verbal fluency as well as to inhibit an overlearned verbal response		
	1. Color labeling	50	Average
	2. Reading words	20	Below average
	3. Inhibition—Label the color of a word printed in a different color than the word	75	High average
	4. Verbal inhibition and cognitive fluency—Requires the individual to switch between reading a color word and labeling the color.	50	Average

(continued)

Table 5-1 (continued).

Psychoeducational Assessment Results

Test Results and Interpretations

Scores are presented in terms of the range they fall into and the percentile rank. A percentile rank refers to how well a student scored relative to same-aged peers. For example, a student who scored at the 72nd percentile can be said to be performing equal to or better than 72% of same-aged peers. Alternatively, it could be stated that the student has only been surpassed by 28% of same-aged peers. Most students' scores will fall in the average range, from the 25th to the 74th percentiles.

Ranges	Percentile Rank
Very superior	At or above the 98th percentile
Superior	91st to 97th percentile
High average	75th to 90th percentile
Average	25th to 74th percentile
Low average	9th to 24th percentile
Borderline/low	2nd to 8th percentile
Extremely low	Below the 2nd percentile

Table 5-2.

Jessica's Initial COPM Results (Productivity Section)

	Productivity Issues Identified by Jessica	Importance	Performance	Satisfaction
1	Needs help with handwriting, class note taking, and test taking	10	3	2
2	Completing assignments in an organized way	9	2	2
3	Managing time for classes and assignments—Getting to classes on time and handing in assignments by due date	8	5	1
4	Needs help with reading and understanding written class resources (e.g., study skills)	8	6	4

short-term memory. Jessica's slow speed in processing print is an area of specific weakness for her. It is likely that she will require accommodations for reading, especially for long durations.

Jessica's visual, as well as verbal, skills are an area of strength for her and this should be considered when making recommendations to support her learning.

Results of Canadian Measure of Occupational Performance and Interview With Jessica and Her Parents

The COPM (Law et al., 2005) is administered to help Jessica identify occupational performance issues, with a focus on her role as a student. Given the focus of this chapter, the results of the COPM are reported for the productivity section only (Table 5-2).

With these occupational issues identified and prioritized, the occupational therapist proceeds to explore PEO elements that are relevant to Jessica's current situation. The following PEO elements were described by Jessica and her parents during the initial interview.

Person

> Jessica is a 17-year-old female who has struggled at school for many years.

> Jessica has a diagnosis of a learning disability, attention deficit disorder (ADD), and mild fine motor impairment.

> Jessica reports difficulty with doing up buttons, zippers, and snaps and opening Ziploc snack bags.

> Jessica reports that her writing and printing tend to be messy, and she makes frequent mistakes when texting on the small buttons of her cell phone.

> Jessica easily converses with the assessor.

> Jessica reports she has no history of mental illness.

> Jessica reports that she often experiences anxiety prior to and during test taking.

> Jessica talks about positive interactions with numerous friends at school and says she enjoys social activities.

> Jessica comments that "everything takes me longer to do, and I am always late with things" (i.e., late for classes, assignments are never done on time, and spends more time studying than with her friends but still does more poorly).

> Jessica reports that she has difficulty planning activities, completing tasks on time, and remembering deadlines.

> Jessica often loses things and makes careless mistakes.

Environment

> Jessica is in her last year of high school.

> The high school is now providing special education supports and accommodations for note taking, assignments, and test taking.

> Jessica is looking forward to transitioning from a high school context to a post-secondary educational facility.

> Jessica is aware that supports and expectations will be different than high school.

> Jessica currently resides with both parents and two older siblings.

> Jessica reports that she feels well supported by her family.

> Jessica's mother and siblings provide support for homework, tracking school assignments, events, and deadlines.

> Jessica is planning to live at home during her time at college.

> Jessica's parents drive her to school and to social and extracurricular events most of the time.

> Jessica reports that she will likely pursue driver training in the future but indicates that she wants to focus on school for now: "Between my parents, my brother, and my friends I most always can find a ride wherever I want to go."

> Jessica has several close friends at school, and they call her regularly to do fun things together outside of school.

Occupation

> Jessica is a high school student in her final year of a public education program.

> Jessica is currently on a modified curriculum as outlined in her IEP (she is taking three-fourths caseload with a number of modifications, including assistance of a part-time educational assistant and extra time for tests).

> This term Jessica's courses include English, religion, and biology.

>> Jessica is a member of the student council at her high school and is on the special events committee.

>> Jessica also reports that she volunteers as a friendly/social visitor at a local nursing home 3 days per month.

>> Jessica does not have a part-time job as her parents want her to focus on her schooling.

>> Jessica reports that she is interested in pursuing a career in the medical field, either as a paramedic or nurse.

An analysis of PEO components indicate that there are areas of strength and areas requiring intervention. Areas of strength relate to the positive, strong fit between Jessica's social skills and the social demands of the school environment. There is also a good fit between Jessica's need for help with homework and transportation to various events and her family's support of these activities. Areas requiring attention by the occupational therapist can be described in terms of a poor PEO fit. There appears to be a poor fit between the cognitive and motor demands of school work and Jessica's current challenges with some cognitive and fine motor skills. It is, therefore, appropriate for the occupational therapist to use a cognitive-neurological approach to guide an in-depth assessment of the underlying components that influence academic performance. It is also possible that the poor fit between Jessica's current skills and the demands of written school tasks are biomechanical in nature. Therefore, a physical approach may be useful to assess ergonomic factors, sitting postures, paper position, pencil grasp, and writing instruments, as well as her muscle strength and endurance during written tasks. Consideration will be given throughout the assessment process to her need for assistive technology.

Occupational Therapy Assessment and Intervention

Guided by a combination of cognitive-neurological and physical approaches, the occupational therapist assesses key performance components that could be affecting her school performance:

>> Personal performance components, such as:

◎ Vision and hearing (whisper test and self-report of visual acuity)

◎ Motor function (manual muscle testing, functional observations of range of motion, and motor coordination during different tasks)

◎ Sensation (response to touch)

◎ Pain (self-report)

◎ Visual motor integration and visual perception (administration of Beery-Butenica Developmental Test of Visual Motor Integration, 5th Edition Revised [Beery & Beery, 2006] [VMI] and the Motor-Free Visual Perception Test [MVPT-3] [Colarusso & Hammill, 2003]).

>> Tests of written communication, including handwriting (quality, speed, and legibility) and keyboarding skills

The occupational therapist also utilizes a dynamic assessment approach (Toglia, Golisz, & Goverover, 2009) to try different pointing devices and assistive technology hardware/software to determine the best solution to compensate for Jessica's weaknesses.

Results of Assessment of Physical and Cognitive Neurological Performance Components

Vision and Hearing

Jessica wears corrective lenses for acuity and is able to read a 10-point font on paper and on a computer screen when wearing her glasses. Her last vision assessment was completed within

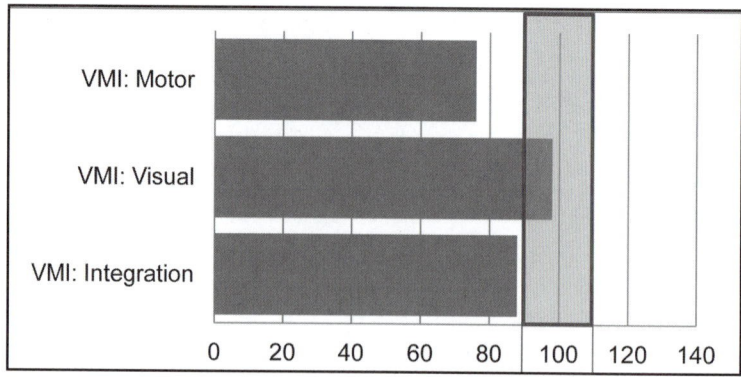

Figure 5-2. Graphic representation of Jessica's results on the Visual Motor Integration measure.

3 months with no recommended changes to her prescription. Hearing is reported to be within normal limits based on a previous hearing assessment.

Upper and Lower Extremity Function

Jessica demonstrated full muscle strength and full range of motion in her upper and lower extremities during task performance. Jessica is right-hand dominant and demonstrates minor impairment in fine motor functioning, which includes difficulty with rapid alternating movements of her digits and imprecise hand-eye coordination. Jessica has no impairments in her lower extremities and reports a sitting tolerance of 1 to 1.5 hours.

» Head, neck, lateral flexion, and trunk control

  ◎ No issues reported or observed

» Sensation

  ◎ This was assessed using application of light touch stimulation of digits bilaterally with eyes closed

  ◎ Jessica's sensation of her upper extremities is intact

  ◎ No sensory processing issues noted during assessment

» Pain

  ◎ Nothing significant reported at the time of assessment

» Visual motor integration and visual perception

  ◎ These performance components are assessed via administration of the visual perceptual assessments listed below

  ◎ A brief description of the assessment tool and a summary of Jessica's performance are provided

Visual-Motor Integration

The VMI (Beery & Beery, 2006) is an individually administered, paper-and-pencil test of visual-motor skills that requires the individual to duplicate several basic geometric figures by drawing them. An individual's performance on this test involves fine motor development, perceptual discrimination skills, and the ability to integrate perceptual and motor processes. Therefore, it involves both perceptual input and motor output. Poor performances on this test may be indicative of perceptual (input) difficulties, fine motor (output) difficulties, and/or problems with integrating these processes. Jessica's results on the VMI are summarized in Figure 5-2.

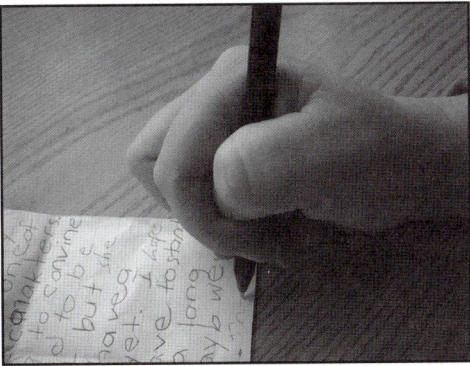

Figure 5-3. Jessica's hand position during handwriting.

The results of the VMI indicate that Jessica presents with below average visual motor integration skills overall. Her visual perception falls in the average range. Jessica's motor coordination appears to fall below the average range. This result is consistent with her self-reported difficulties with fine motor tasks. During the administration of the VMI, Jessica appeared to work on her designs very cautiously. Given that Jessica's motor coordination score is weaker than the visual perception skills on the VMI, it is decided that administration of the MVPT-3 is warranted in order to test the functioning of visual perceptual skills without the influence of her fine motor impairments.

Visual Perception

The MVPT-3 (Colarusso & Hammill, 2003) is an individually administered test designed to assess overall visual perceptual ability in individuals aged 4 to 95 plus years. The MVPT-3 is referred to as motor-free because it does not place any demands on an individual's motor skills. This assessment employs simple black and white drawings as stimulus items. It provides answer choices in a multiple-choice format. The key visual perceptual skills that are assessed within this tool include spatial orientation/relationships, visual discrimination, figure-ground, visual closure, visual memory, and form constancy.

Visual perception is the process on which we depend to accurately interpret and prescribe meaning to visual stimuli. The literature acknowledges that individuals with deficits in visual perception may experience difficulties using the telephone, handling money, locating objects, performing self-care tasks, reading, writing, and/or driving.

Jessica's overall MVPT-3 score falls within the below average range. Observations during this assessment indicate that Jessica has particular difficulty with subtests involving form constancy and visual memory. Based on the results of these two visual perception tests (VMI and MVPT-3), it is believed that Jessica's difficulties with handwriting are due to both visual perception as well as fine motor deficits.

Handwriting Skills

Table height and computer chair are adjusted to ensure optimal ergonomic positioning. A sample of Jessica's handwriting is collected using a timed test. Jessica is first observed to copy a written sample provided to her (copy task) and then to write a paragraph on a topic of her choice (novel composition task).

While writing, Jessica maintains a slightly forward posture using her left forearm on the table for stability. She writes with her right dominant hand using a lateral tripod grasp (Figure 5-3). She stabilizes the paper with her non-dominant hand while writing. Jessica maintains a static

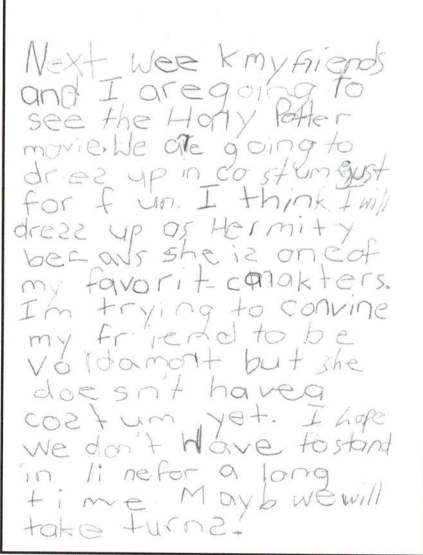

Figure 5-4. Handwriting sample.

wrist flexion and initiates writing from her shoulder, rather than using transitional movements from the intrinsic muscles of her digits. This modified biomechanical presentation is indicative of weak musculature within the hand and minor fine motor impairments. Her writing speed on a 5-minute copy test is an average of 15.0 words per minute (WPM), which is considered to be below her grade level according to most handwriting speed test norms (Honaker, 2003).

An analysis of Jessica's handwriting indicates that she preferred to print and use a gel pen when completing the writing samples. She is able to maintain baseline orientation (i.e., write in a straight line following the lines on the paper) when copying a sample of handwriting and composing her own paragraph. Her writing demonstrates inconsistent pressure, resulting in some words appearing darker and others quite faint. Several spelling errors are noted as well as letter reversals (i.e., backwards letters commonly "r," "h," and "s"). The legibility of her written output is also compromised by inconsistent spacing between words (i.e., some words merging together or excessive gaps between letters within a word). Figure 5-4 offers a sample of her handwriting. These common errors are indicative of poor motor planning, impairments in fine motor control, and an inefficient grasp.

The results of the visual perceptual testing help to further explain some of the issues identified with Jessica's handwriting. For example, she has particular difficulty with the MVPT-3 subtests involving use of form constancy and visual memory. The impairment in these skills are further supported by the letter reversals and spelling errors noted in Jessica's handwriting sample.

It should also be noted that Jessica needs some cueing in helping her to select a topic and initiate writing during the novel composition task. She often re-reads her sentences aloud several times before moving on to writing the next sentence. This presentation is consistent with some of the issues identified in the psychoeducational report (i.e., slow processing and deficits in working memory), as well as Jessica's comments during the interview regarding difficulty with organization and planning.

Additionally, this therapist reviews several of Jessica's completed written assignments and the above, mentioned deficits become more apparent as the complexity of the written task increases, particularly with regards to spelling, planning, and overall organization.

Table 5-3.		
Assistive Technology Trialled in Dynamic Assessment		
Assistive Technology Trialled	**Description**	**Observation and Analysis of Client Performance**
Computer, standard keyboard, and mouse	A desktop computer with current operating system was used to assess Jessica's keyboarding and mouse access	• Legibility of written output while typing was improved compared to handwriting. The typed document demonstrated improvement in visual presentation including improved word spacing, letter formation, and overall spatial organization of the document. • Jessica reported that typing was less effortful and fatiguing than handwriting. • The rate of text output increased by 3 WPM with use of the computer. • These improvements may result from the decreased demand on visual motor integration, spatial processing, and fine motor skills required for handwriting compared to keyboarding.
Word prediction software	Software to provide support with text composition (i.e., spelling) The key features of this include: • Auditory feedback of text as you type and read-back text • Display of a wordlist for a word being typed • Prediction ahead of the next word	• Jessica benefitted from the auditory feedback feature of this software, as her rate of text output increased when compared to her use of a standard keyboard. • Less spelling errors were noted as well as improved quality of written output (spacing, spelling). • She was able to use her strengths in visual recognition to identify the appropriate word from the word list.
Speech recognition (SR) software	• Software that translates spoken word into written text • Some SR software applications also have the added benefit of a read-back feature	• Jessica was able to use her strength in all areas of verbal skills (i.e., verbal recognition, verbal memory, and verbal comprehension) to generate text using speech recognition software. • The read-back feature was also beneficial for her to hear and help identify grammatical and software recognition errors. • SR software provided the most substantial increase in the rate of text output. • Jessica required support to recall basic voice commands for functional and efficient operation of this software. • Visual cues (i.e., a written list of voice commands) were utilized to capitalize on her strengths in visual skills and to compensate for poor memory skills.

(continued)

Table 5-3 (continued).		
Assistive Technology Trialled in Dynamic Assessment		
Assistive Technology Trialled	Description	Observation and Analysis of Client Performance
Visual thinking and learning software; mind mapping software	• Software to help visually organize thoughts and concepts (a thinking and learning tool) • The software allows students to build graphic organizers including concept maps, web mind maps, and idea maps to brainstorm, plan, organize, think, outline, and present	• Jessica had a chance to trial this software within the context of planning for an assignment with her resource teacher. • She found it helpful in organizing her thoughts and have a visual representation (map) of her ideas. • The benefit of this software is likely because it appeals to her visual skills, which are a strength for her.
Professional software for scanning and reading text	• Scan read software is a software that reads scanned or electronic text aloud using synthetic speech • Software options include highlighting of words as they are spoken and addition of auditory and or written notes, etc. This auditory and visual presentation of information helps increase reading, accuracy speed, and comprehension for struggling reader	• Jessica's reading speed and tracking along the line being read was supported with this software. • It helps to support her impairments in reading comprehension. It provides visual cues, which are a strength for Jessica.
Personal digital assistants (PDA)	• These devices allow one to have a portable personal electronic organizer for scheduling events, recording due dates, setting alarms, voice memos, etc.	• This would help Jessica to compensate for impairments in memory, time management, and organization.

Keyboarding Skills

Table height and computer chair are adjusted for ergonomic positioning. Jessica directly accesses the keyboard with bilateral index fingers using a "hunt and peck" method to locate keys. Jessica is able to generate novel text with spelling errors. Keyboarding for written output results in improved legibility of Jessica's text. The fact that legibility of typed text is superior to the handwritten text is likely due to the fact that keyboarding decreases the demands on fine motor skills and visually motor integration. Jessica is able to accurately target the keys on the standard keyboard. She is able to identify and correct errors more consistently when keyboarding.

Five Minute Copy Test: 18 Words-Per-Minute With Spaces

Although Jessica's speed of text composition is only slightly faster via keyboarding (increase of 3 WPM), the quality and legibility of this written output is significantly improved via typing as compared to handwriting.

Dynamic Assessment of Assistive Device Use

A dynamic assessment process is now used with Jessica to determine the best fit between PEO components. The occupational therapist changes one element at a time and observes Jessica's performance (Toglia et al., 2009).

The first assessment is in relation to her use of pointing devices. Jessica is familiar with, and prefers to use, a regular mouse. She has sufficient control to access on-screen targets using the standard mouse. Rate of the double-click function is decreased within the standard Microsoft Windows (Redmond, Washington) accessibility properties. In order to accommodate for fine motor limitations, she is observed functionally using a trackpad mouse built into the standard laptop, with the same modifications made to the double-click speed.

The next part of the dynamic assessment process involves trials of different software. Table 5-3 outlines the different technology that Jessica tried and the observations of the therapist.

The results of the full occupational therapy assessment, including the assistive devices trials, led the occupational therapist to make the specific recommendations to the special education team at her school. The occupational therapist's report included a summary statement:

> *The following academic accommodations for Jessica are recommended in order to help her meet her academic needs and to address the issues that she identified in the occupational therapy assessment. These recommendations include implementation of strategies as well as the use of assistive technologies that will allow Jessica to compensate for areas of weakness and maximize occupational performance in her role as a student.*

The occupational therapist then summarized the recommendations in a table format that was organized around the four occupational issues that Jessica identified in the COPM (Table 5-4). This enables all readers to understand the reasoning of the occupational therapist.

Table 5-4 shows that the recommendations from the occupational therapist include both assistive technology (AT) equipment as well as learning strategies, which makes it easy for school personnel to understand. Funding approval was received by the school, and the equipment was purchased for Jessica.

Intervention continues once weekly for an additional 6 weeks to provide Jessica with assistance for training in the use of speech recognition software (Figure 5-5), mind mapping and organizational software, and the use of the personal digital assistants (PDA). The occupational therapist's skills in educating clients ("Learning through doing" [Townsend et al., 2007]) was critical here.

Jessica's educational assistant is also included in these training sessions and plays an active role in implementation of the learning strategy recommendations. Regular training and support by a qualified professional is an important factor in ensuring that the technology is used appropriately and to prevent abandonment.

The goal of occupational therapy in an academic environment is to improve a student's performance of occupations and tasks that are important for school functioning. Assessment and subsequent recommendations for task adaptations, task modifications, and assistive technology may be necessary to optimize the student's performance in the school setting. The occupational therapist can also play an important role in educating and training the student and school personnel in the use of assistive technology. This enables a student with learning disabilities to prepare for future post-secondary education opportunities.

Conclusion

Prior to Jessica's graduation from high school, the occupational therapist reassesses her occupational performance and written communication skills.

Table 5-4. **Occupational Therapy Recommendations**			
Jessica's Performance Issues From the COPM	Areas Impacting Optimal Performance	Recommended Learning Strategies	Recommended Assistive Technology
Needs help with handwriting (e.g., class note taking, test taking, and homework)	• Difficulty with spelling • Slow reading speed • Slow working memory • Slow processing • Decreased fine motor coordination resulting in slow handwriting speed and poor legibility of written output • Impairments in visual motor integration and visual perception • Therefore, less efficiency in completion of handwriting tasks	• Extra time to complete tests and examinations (50% extra time) • Assistance of a reader on tests and exams that have lengthy reading components • Alternative format of test questions to reduce handwriting requirements and demands on working memory (i.e., multiple choice versus short answer questions) • Oral exams where possible • Record lectures and class sessions • Obtain an electronic copy of class notes	• Writing tests and examinations on a computer with the use of a spell checker and auto-correct options • Use of speech recognition software as an alternative form to handwriting for both homework and test taking • Use of a digital recorder to record and review class sessions
Difficulty completing assignments in an organized way	• Weak organization and self-monitoring skills • Impaired planning and processing abilities • Memory impairments	Prior to writing an assignment, Jessica should: 1. Brainstorm her ideas for her topic 2. Create an outline of the structure of her paper (i.e., subheadings and point form details of what she wishes to discuss) 3. Review and reorganize as necessary 4. Look for spelling and grammatical errors 5. Use color-coding and point form notes when reviewing readings and use resource materials to assist in organizing and processing relevant content	• Use of mind mapping software to facilitate the brainstorming and planning process and to improve organization of completed written work • Electronic copies of class readings and use of many of the reading comprehension software features would allow Jessica to make either recorded notes or text (via dictation with software) notes within the reading materials • The color features of the reading comprehension software would also be useful in organizing these notes

(continued)

Table 5-4 (continued).			
Occupational Therapy Recommendations			
Jessica's Performance Issues From the COPM	Areas Impacting Optimal Performance	Recommended Learning Strategies	Recommended Assistive Technology
Difficulty completing assignments in an organized way			• Integration of the multiple technologies provided • Jessica could then copy relevant color coded notes into the appropriate sub-headings in the mind-mapping software to provide a detailed template that she can then use to write her final assignment • The main goal is to break down the steps involved in completing an assignment and then provide her with the cues and support she needs to complete the process in a step-by-step easy to follow process
Managing time for classes and assignments (e.g., getting to classes and completing assignments by due dates)	• Poor planning and organization (impacting on time management) • Poor attention • Weakness in short-term memory and working memory	• Reduced course-load as needed • Extra time for completion of tests and assignments as needed	• Use of a PDA with an electronic calendar (to record due dates, class times, etc.) and built in alarms to facilitate time management and provide memory cues for completion of tasks or initiation of other actions (i.e., leave for class and begin studying) • Use of speech recognition software will facilitate faster completion of assignments due to increased rate of written output as compared to handwriting

(continued)

Table 5-4 (continued).			
Occupational Therapy Recommendations			
Jessica's Performance Issues From the COPM	**Areas Impacting Optimal Performance**	**Recommended Learning Strategies**	**Recommended Assistive Technology**

Help with reading and understanding written class resources (i.e., study skills)	• Reduced reading speed
	
	• Overall inefficient studying skills due to all of the previous issues mentioned (impaired processing speed, working memory, and visual perceptual issues)
		• Request alternative format for reading materials
		
		• Have a reader to assist with reading components of tests/ examinations
		
		• Introduce study skill strategies to increase efficiency in remembering information and reduce required study time:
		
		  - Allot time for studying and reading every day
		
		  - Review lecture notes and summary notes of reading assignments on a regular basis
		
		  - Minimize last-minute studying
		
		  - Schedule regular breaks into study time (e.g., 10 minutes every 1 to 2 hours)
		
		  - Use calendars to record assignments, organize study time, and daily and weekly activities
		
		• Working in a non-distracting environment
		
		• Determine most productive study time and plan work sessions during that period
		
		• Participate in study groups to discuss or share information regarding what they have read, which may help encourage retention and comprehension
			• Electronic or audio book format of textbooks and class readings
			
			• Reading comprehension software can then be used to read text aloud
			
			• The highlighting, creating written notes/voice notes features within this software can be used to assist with studying and emphasize pertinent information
			
			• Reviewing digital recordings of lectures to increase processing and memory of relevant class information

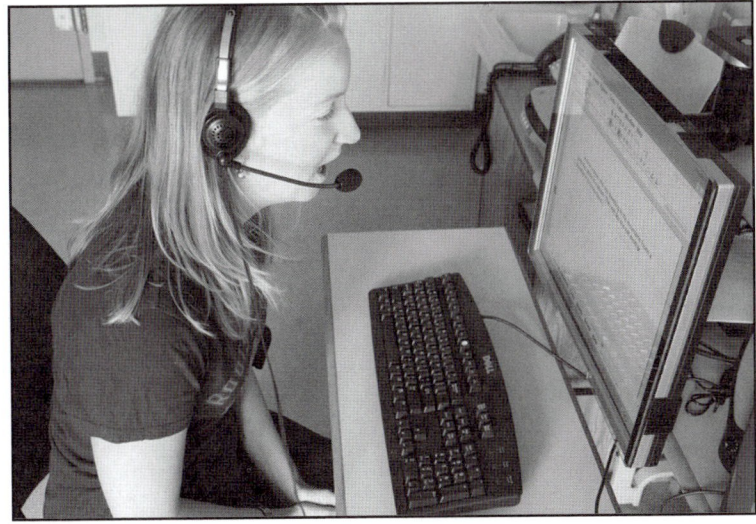

Figure 5-5. Photograph of Jessica taken during a training session using voice recognition software.

Table 5-5.		
Pre- and Post-Intervention Results for Jessica		
	Initial Assessment	**Reassessment**
Handwriting speed	15.0 WPM*	15.2 WPM
Typing speed	18.0 WPM	18.0 WPM
Speech Recognition	26.0 WPM	37.0 WPM
*WPM = words per minute		

Quantitatively, Jessica has shown considerable improvement in her writing speed with use of speech recognition software (see Figure 5-5). The quality of the written output with respect to spelling errors and legibility is also significantly improved. Table 5-5 displays the results for the rate of written output at the time of initial assessment and post-intervention.

The COPM is readministered in order to determine if the technology and strategies in place are helping Jessica to meet her productivity goals with respect to occupational performance as a student (Table 5-6).

Based on the COPM results, as well as Jessica's comments below, implementation of technology and learning strategies and the provision of thorough training and follow-up have helped her to address some of her concerns with respect to her academic performance. The changes in the performance and satisfaction ratings are quite significant.

The Occupational Therapist Received a Note From Jessica 1 Year Later

I was so lucky to get help from you in my last year of high school—the AT you recommended made my grades better than ever. You helped me receive funding that my family did not know I was eligible for, and you helped me purchase equipment, such as the speech recognition software and the training on how to use the software. I can use this software to make notes, to do homework, and to chat with my friends. For once, I can actually get some work done faster than some of my peers.

	Needs Identified	Importance	Performance		Satisfaction	
			Pre	Post	Pre	Post
1	Needs help with handwriting, class note taking, test taking	10	3	7	2	8
2	Completing assignments in an organized way	9	2	6	2	6
3	Managing time for classes and assignments—getting to classes on time and handing in assignments by due date	8	5	8	1	7
4	Help with reading and understanding written class resources (i.e., study skills)	8	6	8	4	7

Table 5-6.

Canadian Occupational Performance Measure Results for Jessica Post-Intervention

I was worried that I might not be able to make it to college, but with my improved grades, I was accepted into the program of my choice. It has been a huge change for me, but I love my classes. I went to the disability office in the summer to meet with a learning specialist—and guess what; she is an occupational therapist, too. She understood everything I told her and knows about the assistive technology I need to use. She is helping me get the accommodations in place here at the college. There are more people to talk to, but I'm doing okay as I understand my disability now and can explain it to others. Thank you again for helping me get the supports and technology I needed to be successful.

Jessica is like many other students with learning disabilities who require ongoing supports to ensure continued success as they make their transition to post-secondary studies. Occupational therapists are well suited to assist with this transition with our unique lens of PEO transactions and our competencies in the analysis and use of occupation, task, and activity. We can also support students in developing self-advocacy skills, which they will need in higher education settings (Hitchings, 2001).

Increasingly, occupational therapists are being drawn to work in this environment to ensure full inclusion and accessibility of higher learning for all. In the post-secondary environment, occupational therapists may work in the disability services and/or accessible learning services departments. Their role in this department is to support human rights legislation, which ensures that students with disabilities have the right to be accommodated. The goal of accommodation is to allow equal benefit from participation and full inclusion (Ontario Human Rights Commission, 2008). There is no set formula for accommodating people with disabilities; therefore, occupational therapists must use their assessment skills and unique clinical reasoning to determine the best fit for each student, including the accommodations and supports that will work best. Ultimately, we can contribute to building capacity for full participation and inclusion of all youth with disabilities, through enabling optimal occupational performance in all environments.

The Higher Education Quality Council of Ontario (Sweet, Anisef, Brown, Adamuti-Trache, & Parekh, 2012) has documented the importance of transition planning in supporting students with special needs who aspire to continue with their education at the post-secondary level. While this document incorporates many individuals with special needs, it also includes individuals with learning disabilities.

The expert panel indicated that there is a paucity of research on the transition of students with special needs between secondary and post-secondary schooling (Sweet et al., 2012).

Inclusive policies at both the school and post-secondary level are designed to encourage students with special needs to continue with their education. However, relatively few do so. Some students with special needs fail to complete their schooling and drop. Others graduate from high school but decide against enrolling in a college or university program. While some of these students may prefer direct entry into the labor others have post-secondary aspirations for which they are not adequately prepared or supported. The social goal of inclusive education is to accommodate the aspirations of all students, including those designated as special needs. The existing research on college and university access suggests that students with special needs who aspire to post-secondary education face significant barriers.

This further supports the importance of the occupation therapy professional perspective as indicated above. Occupational therapists are well suited to assist in identifying barriers that may limit an individual's occupational performance in the academic setting. Similarly, there is a need to maximize the fit of an individual's abilities with post-secondary educational goals, which may include vocational skills training or further pursuit of academic studies. In order to maximize the success of transitional planning for individuals with special needs from high school to post-secondary education, involvement needs to be initiated at the high school entry level and to continue through until the individual is well established in the post-secondary environment.

Review Questions

1. How does the role of the "student" help youth develop independence and interdependence?

2. What are some of the processes that impact learning and academic performance in students with learning disabilities?

3. What are some assistive technology resources and devices that can support students with learning disabilities?

4. How do our roles as occupational therapists make us well-suited to assist youth with disabilities in his or her transition to post-secondary education?

References

Batorowicz, B., Missiuna, C. & Pollock, N (accepted). Technology supporting written productivity in children with learning disabilities: A critical review. *Canadian Journal of Occupational Therapy.*

Beery, K.E., & Beery, N. A. (2006). *The Beery-Butenica development test of visual-motor integration: Administrative, scoring, and teaching manual* (5th ed.). Minneapolis, MN: NCS Pearson.

Chwirka, B., Gurney, B., & Burtner, P. (2002). Keyboarding and visual-motor skills in elementary students: A pilot study. *Occupational Therapy in Healthcare*, 16(2/3), 39-50.

Colarusso, R. P., & Hammill, D. D. (2003). *Motor-free visual perception test* (3rd ed.). Novato, CA: Academic Therapy Publications.

Hitchings, W. E., Luzzo, D. A., Ristow, R., Horvath, M., Retish, P., & Tanners, A. (2001). The career development needs of college students with learning disabilities: In their own words. *Learning Disabilities: Research and Practice*, 16(1), 8-17.

Honaker, D. (2003). *Handwriting speed and legibility literature review*. Retrieved October 31, 2011 from www.fimcvi.org/wp-content/themes/fimcvi/articlepdfs/Cheat_Sheet_Speed_and_legibility_08_03.pdf

Humphry, R. (2009). Occupation and development: A contextual perspective. In E. B. Crepeau, E. S. Cohn, & B. A. Boyt Schell (Eds.), *Willard and Spackman's occupational therapy* (11th ed., pp. 22-32). New York, NY: Lippincott Williams & Wilkins.

Killean, E., & Hubka, D. (1999). *Working towards a coordinated national approach to services, accommodations and policies for post-secondary students with disabilities: Ensuring access to higher education and career training*. Ottawa, Ontario, Canada: National Educational Association of Disabled Students (NEADS).

Law, M., Baptiste, S., Carswell, A., McColl, M. A., Polatajko, H. J., & Pollock, N. (2005). *Canadian Occupational Performance Measure* (4th ed.). Ottawa, Ontario, Canada: CAOT Publications Ace.

Learning Disabilities Association of Canada (LDAC). (2007). *Putting a Canadian face on learning disabilities (PACFOLD)*. Ottawa Ontario, Canada: LDAC.

Learning Disabilities Association of Ontario. (2011). *What are learning disabilities?* Retrieved on October 30, 2011 From http://www.ldao.ca/introduction-to-ldsadhd/introduction-to-ldsadhd/what-are-lds/

Levine, P., & Nourse, S. W. (1998). What follow-up studies say about post-school life for young men and women with learning disabilities: A critical look at the literature. *Journal of Learning Disabilities, 31*(3), 212-233.

McHale, K., & Cermak, S. A. (1992). Fine motor activities in elementary school: Preliminary findings and provisional implications for children with fine motor problems. *American Journal of Occupational Therapy, 46*(1), 898-903.

Mull, C. A., & Sitlington, P. L. (2003). The role of technology in the transition to post-secondary education of students with learning disabilities: A review of the literature. *Journal of Special Education, 37*(1), 26-33.

National Joint Committee on Learning Disabilities. (1990). *Learning disabilities: Issues on definition.* Retrieved October 28, 2011 from www.ldonline.org/about/partners/njcld/archives

Ontario Human Rights Commission. (2008). *Disability and the Duty to accommodate: Your rights and responsibilities.* Retrieved October 30, 2011 from www.ohrc.on.ca/en/issues/disability

Riddell, S., Tinklin, T., & Wilson, A. (2005). *Disabled students in higher education: Perspectives on widening access and changing policy.* New York, NY: Routledge.

Rogers, S. L. (2010). Common conditions that influence children's participation. In J. Case-Smith & N. O'Brien (Eds.), *Occupational therapy for children* (6th ed.) (pp. 146-192). Maryland Heights, MI: Mosby Elsevier.

Schoonover, J., Argabrite Grove, R. E., & Swinth, Y. (2010). Influencing participation through assistive technology. In J. Case-Smith & N. O'Brien. *Occupational therapy for children* (6th ed., pp. 146-192). Maryland Heights, MI: Mosby Elsevier.

Shapiro, B., Church, R. P., & Lewis, M. E. B. (2007). Specific learning disabilities. In M. L. Batshaw, L. Pellegrino, & N. J. Roizen (Eds.), *Children with disabilities* (6th ed., pp. 367-386). Baltimore, MD: Brookes.

Sweet, R., Anisef, P., Brown, R., Adamuti-Trache, M., & Parekh, G. (2012). *Special needs students and transitions to post-secondary education.* Toronto, Canada: Higher Education Quality Council of Ontario.

Toglia, J. P., Golisz, K. M., & Goverover, Y. (2009). Evaluation and intervention for cognitive perceptual impairments. In E. B. Crepeau, E. S. Cohn, & B. A. Boyt Schell (Eds.), *Willard and Spackman's occupational therapy* (11th ed., pp. 739-776). New York, NY: Lippincott Williams & Wilkins.

Townsend, E. A., Beagan, B., Kumas-Tan, Z., Versnel, J., Iwama, M., Landry, J.,...Brown, J. (2007). Enabling: Occupational therapy's core competency. In E. A. Townsend & H. J. Polatajko, (Eds.), *Enabling occupation II: Advancing an occupational therapy vision for health, well-being, and justice through occupation* (pp. 87-133). Ottawa, Ontario, Canada: CAOT Publications ACE.

Townsend, E. A, & Polatajko, H. J. (Eds.). (2007). *Enabling occupation II: Advancing an occupational therapy vision for health, well-being, & justice through occupation.* Ottawa, Ontario, Canada: CAOT Publications ACE.

Vroman, K. (2010). In transition to adulthood: The occupations and performance skills of adolescents. In J. Case-Smith & J. C. O'Brien (Eds.), *Occupational therapy for children* (6th ed.). St. Louis, MO: Elsevier.

Wagner, M., Newman, L., Cameto, R., Levine, P., & Garza, N. (2006). An overview of findings from wave 2 of the National Longitudinal Transition Study-2 (NLTS2). U.S. Department of Education: National Center for Special Education Research.

6

Employment Transitions for Youth With Mental Health Issues

Sandra Moll, PhD, OT Reg (Ont) and Kevin Tregunno

Working represented, for me, a rite of passage… (Kevin Tregunno, May 2011)

The focus of this chapter is on developmental transitions related to employment and how transitions between school and work can be affected by mental illness, and how occupational therapists can support youth during this key time in their development. Many mental health disorders have their onset in late childhood or early adolescence. Whether it is anxiety, depression, substance use, or psychosis, the associated cognitive, emotional, and social problems can have devastating consequences for performance at school and work. Unfortunately, many early intervention programs focus on illness management rather than functional recovery, and as a result, employment needs may not be considered (Rinaldi, 2010; Woodside, Krupa, & Pocock, 2007). Occupational therapists can address this gap in service delivery by advocating for, and supporting youth to achieve their employment goals.

The scenario in this chapter is based on Kevin's journey through adolescence and how involvement in paid employment both shaped and was shaped by his experiences with mental illness. His story serves as a springboard for reflection on how occupational therapists can view his experiences through an occupational therapy lens and how our theoretical approaches can guide our assessments and evidence-based interventions.

It should be noted that much of the research on adolescent employment and mental illness focuses on the population of youth with early psychosis. As such, this is the primary source of evidence-based information in this chapter. Psychosis is a symptom of mental illness in which reality testing may be impaired. Individuals with psychosis may experience hallucinations and/ or distorted ideas, with impaired insight. Since many first episode or early intervention clinics

6

Stewart, D. (Ed.)
Transitions to Adulthood for Youth With Disabilities Through an Occupational Therapy Lens (pp. 103-122).
© 2013 SLACK Incorporated

employ occupational therapists, therapists need to be aware of the key knowledge, skills, and resources needed to work with this population. Also, many of the issues and principles of intervention are relevant to youth with other major mental health disorders.

A Personal Journey Through Adolescence, Work, and Recovery From Mental Illness

My name is Kevin. I am currently 30 years old and have been working in social services for 10 years, including my current position as a peer support provider in an early intervention in psychosis program. My journey to recovery has been shaped in many ways by work-related transitions. I'd like to take you through some of my early experiences with mental illness and explain the role work has played in my recovery, both spiritually and socially.

My early experiences of working were both exciting and challenging. Working represented, for me, a rite of passage and a chance to make extra spending money. It was part of growing up, part of life. As a teenager who was drifting through his high school years with little direction, I got my first job at age 16 as a dishwasher in a fancy downtown restaurant. It was hard work with little pay, but it offered me a chance to connect with society in ways I had not previously experienced.

After about 2 months of slaving in front of a sink and pushing my stress levels to heights I had not known, I quit. It was hard work, but I was also having problems at home, with ongoing bouts of prolonged sadness and difficulties sleeping. My difficulties had gone untreated throughout my teenage years. I was a youth who was having difficulties, both mentally and spiritually. My circle of friends helped me get by, though some of them were troubled as well, and most of them used drugs and drank on weekends. It all seemed so much like the normal thing to do, but it only served to precipitate my problems and make them worse.

In my years prior to high school, my grandma worked at the local department store and would always bring us to the cafeteria during her lunch breaks. The store had certain nostalgic qualities for me, so I jumped at the chance of applying for a job in the same department store they were building in the east part of the city. At age 17, I applied and got a job as cashier.

The most significant thing I can remember about the job is the social aspect, and how the store was filled with people close to my age. I made friends and felt supported there. Despite the challenges, I found it a good test of my capacity for stress, and it even helped me to stay less focused on my depression. It also helped me to get better sleep because I would come home from work and feel exhausted. I worked at that job for almost a year, which I felt was a milestone given I didn't last that long at my first job.

There were many problems going on at home. My mom was struggling with a drinking problem and depression. Our small family was constantly fighting and arguing, so being at home was very stressful and difficult. I enjoyed working because it helped me forget about those problems and offered me an escape. It also gave me something to talk about with my friends like, "today at work some guy…" Work offered me a healthy chance to individuate and experience independence and adulthood. I still had no idea what I wanted to do with my life, but at the time it didn't matter.

It was not until my senior year that I began to feel worried that I had a very uncertain future, with little promise of success. The end of school was approaching fast and I didn't know what I'd do. During one of my grade 12 classes near the end of my high school term, a teacher called me aside and asked me if I'd like to mentor a younger student who was dealing with isolation and having difficulties in school. I agreed to meet with him, kind of shocked that I was even asked. I was a troubled kid myself; I didn't really excel at anything in school, why did she ask me? Little did I know that this was a pivotal moment that would shape my future career direction.

There was a major interruption though, months later, after graduating high school. It came on gradually, and maybe I was too troubled for anyone to see the difference, but I developed psychosis at age 19 and was subsequently diagnosed with schizophrenia. It felt like my whole system, including my mind, was in shock and the side effects of the meds made me stiff. I also could not think straight at times, and I found it hard to even express how I felt. My friends starting treating me differently after I was diagnosed; I was no longer just another normal teen.

My initial reaction of the experience was shock, as I slowly came back to reality in the hospital, with the help of antipsychotics. Yep, life had changed completely now. Or had it? During my stay at the hospital I was baffled, not knowing what had happened or what it would mean for me. I felt my innocence was taken from me by the strange and unreal experience of hallucinations and delusions. It was actually the recreation therapist who helped me the most while I was in there. She woke me up everyday and encouraged me to play games with the groups, do art, listen to music, and just try and make fun out of a terrible situation.

As I slowly recovered and was released to go home, I was encouraged to apply for welfare and then Ontario disability support, but I didn't make it to the orientation. My mom, who I was living with at the time, came down hard on me, stating that if I didn't get a job I'd be kicked out of the house.

I tried temp agencies, but I just couldn't handle the stress. On two different occasions, I came home and told my mom I quit, and she would tell me to get out there and keep trying. I saw an ad on a bus for a program called Job Connect, a job-finding program for youth, and I called them. They gave me a lead on a job at a department store, working as a janitor. I applied and got the job. Shortly after that, I moved out and rented a room with the money I was making. This was 6 months after I had been hospitalized. The job was full time, and it was not easy to get up everyday and do the work. But there was something different about this job, because my boss took special interest in helping me. He talked to me during my shift by phone, sometimes for 30 minutes at a time, and he encouraged a family ethic with me and all my coworkers. It wasn't long before I opened up and told him I had a mental illness. He told me he too had experienced mental illness, and it was nothing to be ashamed of.

As the months went by, I did find it challenging to stay busy at work. Because I worked independently, I often could go off for long periods of time with no one noticing. Sometimes I slept for an hour here and there or went on long lunch breaks. Luckily for me, I was alone most of the time and my thinking didn't cause any problems.

After seeing first-hand what it was like to support myself on a minimum wage job, I realized I wanted to go to school. Having left my old high school drug-using buddies behind and having met a new circle of friends, I found myself feeling renewed and healthier. With the help of my friends, I applied to college for what else? A-ha! Recreation therapy!

In my first year of college, which was exactly 1 year after being diagnosed with schizophrenia, I found school gelled well with where I was at in my life. The classes were interesting, and the people were all accepting and nice. I confided in one of my teachers about my mental illness and was met with acceptance and compassion. She suggested I apply to the disability office to help students with similar problems. So I did.

My first job with the disability office was to mentor a student in my class who had a learning disability. He was a sweet and kind man who didn't have many friends in the class, so I'd sit and study with him. While doing that and studying, I was living on my own. There was a favored pizza shop nearby, which I frequented, and one day, out of the blue, the owner asked if I'd like a job there. So, I took the job. I worked two jobs and went to school full time. Slowly things were coming together. The next year I was asked by the disability office to work with another student who had a learning disability, but this time they doubled my pay.

To see what I was capable of amazed me, and I found myself feeling like I could do anything. I felt so good that I thought I didn't need take my medication, so I went off my antipsychotics and got really ill.

After the smoke cleared from that hospitalization, I finished school and found work at a local coffee shop, where I worked full time. I couldn't find a job as a recreation therapist, and I was feeling very discouraged. I started volunteering at local mental health agencies, and eventually got a break and was hired at a hospital as a peer support worker. After that, things just kept getting better. I shared speech after speech about my experiences, and I won an award for my work. It seemed like things had cleared, and I had begun to realize my calling to a greater extent.

The rest, as they say, is history...

Kevin's Story Through an Occupational Therapy Lens

Occupation, Spirituality, and Development

One of the central developmental tasks of adolescence is to establish a sense of self through considering roles that one will play in the adult world. Erikson, for example, argued that the ages of 14 through 24 years represent a stage where youth acquire a sense of identity through recognition of abilities, interests, strengths, and weaknesses of the self and others (Case-Smith & O'Brien, 2010). Youth begin to develop an occupational identity as part of the process of reflecting on who they are, how they fit in society, and where their lives are headed. Employment represents a socially valued role that can lead to positive outcomes in terms of identity, self-esteem, and social integration (Woodside et al., 2007).

Kevin's story illustrates the many dimensions of meaning that work may have during adolescence and young adulthood. He reflected on his life as a teenager "drifting through high school with little direction," and the role that work played in providing structure, routine, and a way to connect with society. He explained, for example, that work represented "a rite of passage" and "a healthy chance to individuate and experience independence and adulthood." These comments speak to the importance of work in this stage of development. As he neared the end of high school, the anxiety he described regarding his future is not unlike many adolescents who feel pressured to develop an occupational identity and who may be uncertain about their future career directions.

The onset of mental ill health at this critical developmental stage can disrupt functioning at school and work, thereby compromising development of a positive occupational identity and healthy career trajectory (Brown, 2011). The onset of a first episode of psychosis, for example, is frequently associated with a pronounced decline in education and employment (Goulding, Chien & Compton, 2010; Kessler, Foster, Saunders, & Stang, 1995). It has been reported that 50% of young people with psychosis have less than 10 years of education, which then limits their prospects for employment (Killackey, Jackson, & McGorry, 2008). By the time youth come into contact with mental health services, approximately 50% to 70% of individuals with a first episode of psychosis are unemployed, and these unemployment rates rise dramatically within the first few years of treatment (Killackey, Jackson, Gleeson, Hickie, & McGorry, 2006; Singh et al., 2000). Low expectations and lack of support from family and health professionals can contribute to the poor employment rates (Rinaldi et al., 2010).

There are competing ideas noted in the literature about whether work is a benefit or risk to mental health. Mortimer and Staff (2004) reviewed the concerns of prominent developmental psychologists regarding the impact of early employment on the mental health of teens. Concerns have been expressed regarding the time commitment associated with work, indicating that this may restrict opportunities for youth to explore alternative identities and interests and disrupt development of supportive relationships with parents and peers (Greenberger, 1988). Concerns have also been expressed regarding the potential links between work and unhealthy lifestyles, such as increased substance use (Carriere, 2005; Godley, Passetti, & White, 2006). Exposure to older coworkers, the stress of work, and increased access to the means to purchase substances are some of the identified work-related risks for substance use (Godley, et al., 2006; McMorris &

Uggen, 2000; Mortimer & Staff, 2004). Similar concerns were noted in the Canadian report on Improving the Health of Young Canadians (Canadian Institute for Health Information [CIHI], 2005). Findings from the section on employment and working conditions indicated that adolescents who work 20 hours a week or more report higher levels of emotional distress and do not do as well academically. Students who work are also more likely than nonworking students to smoke and regularly consume alcohol (CIHI, 2005). Mental health professionals, in particular, are often concerned about the potential stress of work and whether it might increase the risk of relapse among youth with mental health issues (Rinaldi et al., 2010).

Despite these expressed concerns, there is a growing body of evidence on the importance of work as a key element in the process of recovery. First-person accounts and qualitative studies of persons with a first episode of psychosis echo the themes in Kevin's story about the importance of work, despite illness. The aspirations of young people, regardless of health status, are similar: to have a good place to live, a car to drive, a meaningful relationship, and a job or career (Rinaldi et al., 2010). Finding work is reported to be part of the search for meaning and identity that is central to the recovery process (Killackey, 2010; Ryan, Marshall, Thorburn, LeDrew, & Hogan, 2006). Furthermore, maintaining work represents normality. The sense of belonging and social acceptance that can be obtained through work is particularly important for adolescents (Perry, Taylor, & Shaw, 2007). Adopting the role of worker means being recognized as a contributing member of society and the opportunity to be financially self-sufficient (Perry et al., 2007). A qualitative study by Gioia and Brekke (2003) found that earning an income was believed to be associated with a more positive self-image, greater well-being, and a better quality of life. Iannelli and Wilding (2007) explored the effect of productive activities on young adults (ages 18 to 25) with mental illness. Participants in this phenomenological study reported that engaging in productive occupation strengthened a sense of responsibility, identity, and self-worth. In addition, involvement in these occupations resulted in a sense of building a positive future for the participants. Work, therefore, has multiple, yet powerful, dimensions of meaning for youth who may be experiencing mental health issues.

Kevin's story illustrates how the trajectories of work and mental illness are intertwined. He acknowledged that work was stressful at times, but also important in maintaining his health. He described work as "a good test of my capacity for stress," a way to escape problems at home, and even improve his sleep. Unfortunately, the "major interruption" of illness that he experienced after high school and the subsequent flare up of psychosis in college were difficult points in his life. It took time to recover from those episodes. He did, however, recover and felt that work played a pivotal role in this process and ultimately to the development of a positive occupational identity. Kevin's journey is unique, yet it illustrates how one's story changes over time in response, not only to the trajectory of illness, but also to the social environment at home and at work. Transitions between school, hospital, and work may present both opportunities and challenges (Figure 6-1).

Person-Environment-Occupation Analysis and Theoretical Approaches

Occupational therapists bring a unique theoretical understanding of the opportunities and challenges of employment for youth with mental health issues. A person-environment-occupation (PEO) analysis framework can be applied to pinpoint the source of occupational performance issues and the changes that may need to be made to optimize the fit between the person (worker), the occupation (work), and the environment (workplace).

Many traditional approaches to vocational rehabilitation focus primarily on the worker, examining whether he or she has the skills and abilities to perform the job. A PEO perspective, however, adds depth of understanding and opens possibilities for change. Instead of labeling a worker as either fit or unfit to work, consideration is given to the match between the worker's skills and the requirements of the job and the match between the worker and the demands of the work environment (Cockburn, Kirsh, Krupa, & Gewurtz, 2004). The therapist's role may be to identify supports

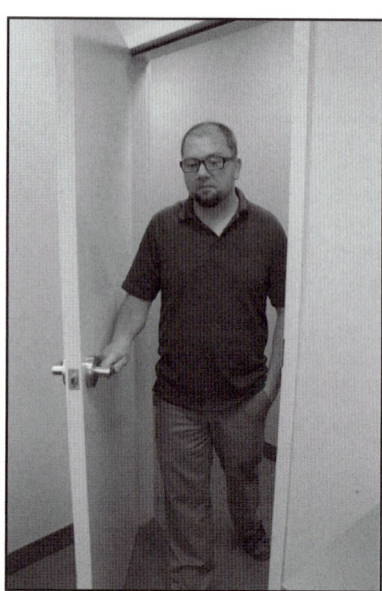

Figure 6-1. Transitions between school, hospital, and work may present both opportunities and challenges.

that can be put in place to optimize the fit between the worker's skills, the job requirements, and the demands of the workplace. If, for example, a client is struggling with social anxiety in an office environment, occupational therapists may help the client to learn skills to cope with his or her anxiety. Skill development, however, may take time. In the meantime, we could explore supports that could be put in place based on an analysis of the social demands of the job and the workplace environment. Optimizing work performance might include consideration of technology to change the job demands (e.g., videoconference attendance at meetings) or arranging for a mentor to provide social support at work. Workplace accommodations that minimize triggers to social anxiety are a way of increasing the fit between the client, the job, and the work environment, thereby supporting the client's ability to function at work.

If we consider the job that Kevin had as a janitor in a department store, his success can be explained from a PEO fit perspective. At the time, Kevin was struggling with motivation, physical fatigue, and disturbing thoughts. Fortunately, the job itself was not beyond his physical abilities, the social and cognitive demands were low, and the independent nature of the work enabled him to take the breaks that he needed. In addition, the social environment was very positive, with a boss who was supportive and encouraging, maintaining regular connections over the phone. Although the PEO fit was perhaps not optimal, it was certainly conducive to maintaining an acceptable level of work performance. This example illustrates the importance of looking beyond individual functioning and considering the client's abilities within the context of job demands and supports. Kevin's story also illustrates that employment is not something that happens at a single point in time, but evolves over time in response to changes in symptoms, occupational demands, and the social environment both within and outside of work. This PEO analysis with Kevin clearly guides the occupational therapist to select a psychoemotional approach to assessment and intervention.

The PEO perspective is a valuable lens to use when considering work transitions for youth with mental health issues. It is important to note that this occupational therapy lens is also compatible with theoretical perspectives outside of the profession. Key perspectives in the mental health field include psychosocial rehabilitation and the recovery model. A 2009 special issue of the *Psychiatric Rehabilitation Journal* profiled the ways in which occupational therapy is positioned in the field of psychosocial rehabilitation. Brown (2009), for example, argues that the basic orientation of occupational therapy and psychiatric rehabilitation are similar, "when considering service provision to support successful and satisfying engagement in everyday life" (p. 162). She also asserts that both orientations use a combination of accommodations, supports, compensatory strategies, and skills training, often in natural environments. Similarly, Krupa, Fossey, Anthony, Brown, and Pitts (2009) describe the compatibility between occupational therapy and psychiatric rehabilitation, including a focus on the person and the environment, the importance of doing in daily life, and a client-centered approach to intervention. They argued that the philosophical foundations of occupational therapy are also consistent with the elements of recovery, such as partnership-centered approaches, renewing hope, moving beyond illness to construct a new self, fostering personal control and responsibility, expanding social roles, and facilitating meaningful community participation. Employment, in particular, is considered to be one of the most important factors in promoting recovery (Rinaldi et al., 2010). The key principles of psychosocial rehabilitation and recovery are central to the process of occupational therapy intervention.

Occupational Therapy Assessment and Intervention

Addressing the employment needs of youth with mental illness and addictions issues should be theoretically informed, yet also supported, by research evidence. Supported employment (SE) is recommended as the current best practice approach for addressing the work issues and goals of individuals with mental illness (Bond, 2004). In particular, the Individual Placement and Support (IPS) model of supported employment (SE) is backed by the most research evidence (Bond, Drake, & Becker, 2008). Unlike traditional vocational interventions that often involve a lengthy period of assessment and prevocational preparation, the IPS model advocates for rapid placement into competitive job positions. The IPS "place then train" approach has consistently led to better employment outcomes, even among youth with mental health disorders (Rinaldi et al., 2010). The focus of this section will therefore be on IPS intervention strategies, including (a) principles of SE, (b) evidence supporting this approach, (c) compatibility with occupational therapy, (d) approaches to assessment, and (e) key intervention strategies.

Principles of Supported Employment

The individual placement and support model was developed in the early 1990s by authors Becker and Drake. As outlined in their training manual, the goal of IPS is "to enable people with mental illness to gain competitive employment in integrated settings with follow-along supports" (Becker & Drake 1993, p. 1). The original manual, entitled *A Working Life: The Individual and Support (IPS) Program* (Becker & Drake, 1993), was recently updated, entitled *Supported Employment: Applying the (IPS) Model to Help Clients Compete in the Workforce* (Swanson & Becker, 2011). The updated manual outlines seven main principles of the IPS model that are central to evidence-based implementation:

1. The first principle, zero exclusion, means that all clients who want to participate are eligible, regardless of their diagnosis, level of wellness, use of substances, work history, or functional impairments.

2. The second principle of IPS is integration of employment and mental health services. Within the IPS model, employment specialists (the vocational service providers) are part of the mental health treatment team and collaborate directly with clinicians providing mental health services. Ongoing formal and informal communication between all team members working with the individual is considered to be an essential part of the service provision.

3. The third principle, competitive employment, is the primary goal of the program. Competitive employment means either part-time or full-time work in the community at a competitive wage in a position that is open to all people, rather than a position reserved for people with disabilities. Volunteer work or employment in sheltered work settings would not be acceptable outcomes within this model.

4. The fourth principle is that of benefits planning, since many clients are afraid of losing their disability and medication benefits if they obtain paid work. Therefore, education and support regarding the implications of work on disability benefits are often needed.

5. The fifth principle, rapid job search, asserts that the job finding phase should occur as soon as possible, avoiding a lengthy process of vocational assessment and/or prevocational training. This principle is based on a philosophy that clients do not want to have to prove their ability to work; instead, their strengths should be recognized and a hopeful attitude communicated regarding everyone's ability to work. It is recommended that the job search process begin within the first month following acceptance into the program.

6. The sixth principle is that of follow-along supports. Follow-along supports are individualized to the client and may include on- or off-site supports (e.g., a job coach). This way the client can access support at any time, even long after he or she starts working. On average, IPS services continue for a year after starting work. Advocacy, education, or counselling is provided, not only to find work, but also to maintain employment over time.

7. The final principle of the IPS model is that client preferences are honored. Rather than linking clients to existing agency jobs or jobs that are readily available in the community, each client's unique interests and goals are identified. Attention to client preferences includes consideration, not only of the client's job-related goals, but preferences regarding service provision (e.g., nature of support provided and decisions about disclosure).

In addition to the key principles, implementation standards have been developed in conjunction with fidelity measures to assess the extent to which the program meets the standards. There are, for example, specific guidelines regarding staffing, organization, and services (Becker, Torrey, Toscano, Wyzick, & Fox, 1998). The manual, fidelity scale, and staff training procedures have been developed to promote standard implementation of IPS services and, therefore, maximize effectiveness of the IPS approach (Swanson & Becker, 2011).

Evidence of Effectiveness

There is evidence from multiple systematic reviews conducted over the past decade regarding the effectiveness of SE, especially the IPS model, for clients with mental health and addictions issues. Crowther, Marshall, Bond, and Huxley (2001) conducted a systematic review of studies comparing SE with prevocational training and concluded that participants in SE programs earned significantly more money and worked more hours per month than clients in prevocational training. A more recent systematic review by Bond and colleagues (2008) included 11 randomized control trials that examined the impact of programs with high fidelity to the IPS model. They concluded that participants in the IPS program had significantly higher rates of competitive employment (61% for the IPS group compared to 23% for controls), took a shorter length of time to find a job (10 weeks earlier than controls), and had a longer job duration (average 24 weeks for the first job).

In addition to studies specifically exploring the IPS approach to SE, there is increasing evidence that the results for the IPS model are stronger when paired with cognitive skills training and social skills training. Executive functioning is a strong predictor of occupational status for individuals with a first episode of psychosis (Dickerson et al., 2008). A randomized control trial conducted by

McGurk, Mueser, Feldman, Wolfe, and Pascaris (2007) compared participants in an SE program with a cognitive training component, "Thinking Skills for Work," with participants in an SE program alone. Follow-up 2 to 3 years later showed that participants in SE plus cognitive training were more likely to work, to be employed for more hours, to be working over a longer period of time, and to earn more than those in the SE-alone program. There is also evidence that social skills training programs tailored to the work environment, when paired with follow-up contact or SE, are effective for improving work outcomes (Mueser et al., 2005; Tsang, Chan, Wong, & Liberman, 2009; Tsang & Pearson, 2001). Nuechterlein et al. (2008a) conducted a randomized control trial comparing an IPS approach plus a social skills program with traditional vocational rehabilitation. Upon 18 months of follow-up, the education and employment rates among IPS clients were twice as high as the group receiving traditional vocational rehabilitation (82% versus 40%). These combinations of IPS with cognitive and social skills programming appears to provide the scaffolding for increased participation in productive occupations (Arbesman & Logsdon, 2011).

Most of the SE research has been conducted with a population of individuals with a severe and persistent mental illness. Rinaldi and colleagues (2010), however, reviewed seven studies that focused specifically on vocational intervention with young adults who experienced a first episode of psychosis. They noted that many of the studies adapted the interventions to include support to fulfill educational goals as well as employment goals, since this is an important priority for many young people. They noted that the education and employment outcomes were particularly positive for studies employing an IPS approach. Across the five IPS studies, the employment and education rate was 69% for IPS versus 35% for the control groups. These outcomes were also reportedly sustained through 6 to 24 months of follow-up (Rinaldi et al., 2010).

Not only do IPS services lead to increased education and employment rates, there is evidence regarding cost effectiveness as well. It has been reported that mental health service costs over a 10-year period were 50% lower for people supported through IPS as compared to other client groups (Bush, Drake, Xie, McHugo, & Haslett, 2009).

Occupational Therapists as Supported Employment Providers

It should be noted that the IPS model is not occupational therapy specific, and the vocational specialists who provide the service are not linked to any particular profession. It has been argued, however, that occupational therapists have a strong foundation of knowledge and skills that position them to be excellent providers of IPS services (Moll, Huff, & Detwiler, 2003). The principles of IPS, for example, are compatible with the values and philosophy of occupational therapy, particularly the emphasis on client preferences, individual strengths, and the importance of meaningful occupation (Auerbach, 2001). We are able to integrate both mental health and vocational interventions, considering symptoms; medication management; and the cognitive, social and emotional effects of mental illness on vocational functioning, as well as job skill development, job accommodations, and career planning. Our expertise in occupational analysis can facilitate the process of job development and provision of follow-along supports (Moll et al., 2003). Job development, for example, involves analyzing potential job opportunities to identify ones that match a client's skills and abilities, as well as his or her preferences (Swanson & Becker, 2011). Provision of follow-along supports involves analysis of each position to identify potential work or workplace modifications that will optimize performance. Gutman, Kerner, Zombek, Dulek, and Ramsey (2009) assert that occupational therapy practitioners have expertise in designing compensatory strategies and accommodation based on individual needs, using activity analysis to break down skills so that they can be gradually mastered, and helping people resume past roles or assume new ones. As outlined earlier, our perspective on the fit between PEO is a key part of this process. Other skills that we bring to the SE process include our ability to build therapeutic partnerships with clients,

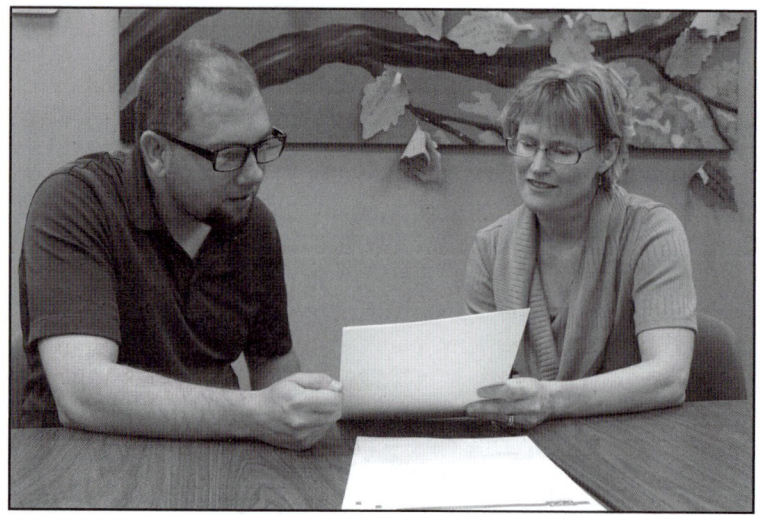

Figure 6-2. The occupational therapist and client meet in partnership to determine client-centered goals.

engage in problem solving, advocate for client needs, and enable clients to advocate for themselves (Moll et al., 2003). We are able to establish effective partnerships to enable change (Figure 6-2).

Although occupational therapists have a strong foundation of skills, providing SE services may require some additional skill development. In order to be effective employment specialists, for example, we need to be able to not only work with individual clients, but to link with employers in the community. Networking with prospective employers is a key part of creating or finding job matches. Marketing clients to potential employers and negotiating workplace supports is also a key part of the process. This involves developing a good understanding of the employer's perspective and creating a "business case" for change (Moll et al., 2003; Porteous & Waghorn, 2009). Job developers need to be out in the community talking with employers in a language that they can understand, and discussing the ways in which clients can address their unique needs (Luecking, 2008). It is important to be persistent since rejection is common, as in anyone's job search. We need to have strong advocacy skills and to consider the needs, goals, and abilities of the individual client, as well as the perspectives and roles of various stakeholders in the workplace (e.g., managers, human resource staff). We must also be aware of relevant legislation governing disability and work (Stergiou-Kita, Moll, Walsh, & Gewurtz, 2010). For occupational therapists new to the role of job development, it may be helpful to consult texts such as *The Job Developer's Handbook: Practical Tactics for Customized Employment* (Griffin, Hammis & Geary, 2007) or *Demystifying Job Development: Field-Based Approaches to Job Development for People With Disabilities* (Hoff, Gandolfo, Gold, & Jordan, 2000) for practical tips and strategies.

Since SE is currently one of the most effective models of enabling individuals to achieve their employment goals, we need to be knowledgeable about the approach, critically reflect on the ways that we provide vocational services, and challenge ourselves to change if our current methods are not consistent with the evidence in the literature.

Assessment Approaches in Supported Employment

Occupational therapists are often asked to conduct vocational assessments to determine whether an individual has the prerequisite knowledge, skills, and abilities for competitive employment. In fact, there may be a range of work-related barriers for youth with mental health issues ranging from active symptomatology, to limited social skills, to lack of work experience (Bell & Lysaker, 1995; Kirsh, 2000). There may be questions about whether the client is ready for work.

As outlined earlier, the emphasis of SE is on a rapid job search, rather than extensive prevocational assessment. In fact, assessment in this model is framed as a continuous process rather than something that happens exclusively prior to the job search (Swanson & Becker, 2011). There is no determination of whether or not a client is ready to work, but rather an opportunity to enable him or her to develop his or her skills and abilities over time (Swanson & Becker, 2011).

At the initial stage in the process, however, there is some basic information that needs to be gathered. Swanson and Becker (2011) describe the importance of developing a career profile that considers the client's work goal, his or her educational and work history, work-related skills and resources, approach to managing illness, and potential network of contacts for the job search. This profile can be expanded upon over time and may involve consultation (with permission) with family members, previous employers, and other members of the treatment team.

Assessment of aptitudes, preferences, and the fit between the individual and the work environment are considered to be important, but conceptualized as an ongoing process rather than something that is completed prior to finding work. Each competitive employment position is considered to be an opportunity to learn more about the client's work abilities and challenges. As part of this ongoing assessment process, barriers or challenges to optimal job performance should be identified as they relate to the worker, work, or workplace environment.

Assessment of the "worker" includes consideration of his or her skills or abilities and impairments, as well as his or her perceptions of the job and work environment. Predictors of success in SE include the motivation and self-efficacy of the worker (Bond et al., 2001; MacDonald-Wilson, Rogers, & Anthony, 2001). In fact, these personal qualities are reported to have more of an impact on vocational outcomes than symptomatology (Rinaldi et al., 2010). It may, therefore, be important to initially understand the client's motivation to work. Decisional balance tools for example, may facilitate an understanding of any ambivalence to pursuing employment (Graham, Jutla, Higginson, & Wells, 2008). Motivational interviewing strategies could then be utilized to build readiness for change. A good employment history is also a strong predictor of successful work outcomes (Poon, Siu, & Ming, 2010). One example of a standardized tool that could be used to gather information from the client is the Worker Role Interview, a tool developed by proponents of the Model of Human Occupation (Pitts, 2011). This interview tool is designed to be utilized at an initial stage of gathering information about the client's perceptions of abilities and limitations, commitment to the worker role, perception of the impact of illness on nonwork roles, ability to adjust habits and routines, and perceptions of the work environment (Braveman et al., 2005). Other performance-based tools that have been reported to have reasonable validity and clinical utility with a mental health population include the Assessment of Work Performance (Sandqvist, Bjork, Gullberg, Henriksson, & Gerdie, 2009) and the Assessment of Motor and Process Skills (Haslam, Pepin, Bourbonnais, & Grignon, 2010). It should be noted, however, that the SE approach is based on ongoing "on the job assessment" of performance, rather than something that is done outside of the context of work. Situational assessments are, therefore, a preferred approach for assessing work function in the mental health field (Pitts, 2011). The Work Behavior Inventory is one example of a situational assessment tool that was developed to measure on-site work performance of persons with psychiatric disabilities (Bryson, Bell, Lysaker, & Zito, 1997). Bryson and colleagues (1997) explain that the tool consists of five behavioral scales (work habits, work quality, personal presentation, social skills, and cooperativeness) that lead to a global rating of work behavior. Ratings are based on a combination of a 10- to 15-minute observation of in vivo work performance and a semistructured interview with the worksite supervisor. Concurrent validity, interrater reliability, and discriminant validity have been demonstrated in several studies (Bryson et al., 1997; Bryson, Bell, Greig, & Kaplan, 1999).

Assessment of the work involves conducting a job demands analysis to identify risk factors as well as "opportunities to adjust or alter workstations, work procedures, processes, or tools to minimize physical and cognitive/emotional strain" (Lysaght, Shaw, Almas, Jogia, & Lamour-Trode, 2008, p. 12). An understanding of the job requires an understanding of (a) essential job duties,

(b) work demands (e.g., physical, cognitive, communication, psychosocial, and behavioral), (c) performance expectations (e.g., quality, quantity, and speed), (d) limitations that may affect work performance (e.g., impairments and balance between home and work demands), and (e) strategies that may enhance work performance (Stergiou-Kita et al., 2010). A job demands analysis can also be used to identify job barriers and facilitators relative to individual functioning and to highlight potential work accommodations that could support work performance. The City of Toronto Job Demands Analysis is a promising tool that can measure cognitive and behavioral work demands (Lysaght et al., 2008). This tool includes 17 cognitive and behavioral items measuring a range of potential job demands (e.g., memory, attention to detail, deadline pressures, and need to work cooperatively with others). The perceived demand for each item is rated using a 4-point ordinal scale. There is emerging evidence regarding the reliability and validity of this tool (Lysaght et al., 2008).

Assessment of the work environment is an additional consideration in the PEO analysis process. There are many studies exploring psychosocial risk factors in the workplace and the impact of job stress on mental health. Sources of job-related stress include not only the content of work (e.g., workload and lack of meaning), but also the context of the work environment (e.g., job insecurity, lack of control over work, and interpersonal conflict) (Harnois & Gabriel, 2002). The social context of the work environment can be a particular challenge for youth with mental health issues, since social participation is often disrupted. Conversely, social support in the workplace can have a significant positive impact on employment outcomes (Rinaldi et al., 2010). Exploring perceptions of stressors and supports in the workplace may therefore be an important part of the assessment process. Pitts (2011) suggests two standardized tools that could be used to explore client perceptions of the work environment, the Work Environment Impact Scale (WEIS) and the Work Environment Scale. The WEIS is a semistructured interview that can be used to explore the client's perception of the physical, social, and temporal aspects of his or her current work environment. The client then rates the degree to which the specific aspects of the environment either support or interfere with his or her success and satisfaction at work (Moore-Corner, Kielhofner, & Olson, 1998). The Work Environment Scale is a 90-item self-report instrument that focuses on client perceptions of the social environment at work (Moos, 1994). These standardized tools may be used when you want to gather detailed information about the client's perceptions of specific aspects of the work environment.

Intervention Strategies

There are a range of work-related challenges experienced by youth with mental health issues that may need to be addressed in order to support their success at work. MacDonald-Wilson, Rogers, and Massaro (2003) outlined the key physical, cognitive, emotional, and social limitations that may be experienced by individuals with psychiatric disabilities. Physical limitations include poor stamina; the pace of work may be slow and more breaks may be required. Cognitive limitations may impair a client's ability to concentrate, process and respond to instructions, learn new tasks, solve problems, plan and organize work, make decisions, follow a schedule, and assess his or her own work performance. Emotional limitations may include difficulty in managing stress and time pressures, regulating emotions (e.g., expressing anger and dealing with disappointment), adjusting to changes in work demands, and displaying confidence in oneself and one's work abilities. Social limitations may include difficulty in communicating with supervisors (e.g., clarifying instructions, asking questions, and asking for help), socializing with coworkers, responding to feedback/criticism, and interpreting social cues (e.g., maintaining boundaries of personal space and choosing conversation topics). In addition to the illness-related challenges, youth with mental health issues may have a limited work history. Lack of previous work experience may mean that they have limited awareness of the expectations for performance at work. It may take time to adjust to work routines and expectations.

Some of the challenges identified above may be addressed through skills training. As outlined earlier, there are cognitive and social skills training programs that could be provided in conjunction with SE (as opposed to a prevocational training program) (McGurk et al., 2007; Nuechterlein et al., 2008b). Motivational interviewing approaches could also be incorporated to address ambivalence that the client may have regarding work (Graham et al., 2008). The primary emphasis in SE is on providing supports or accommodations in the workplace to enable the client to be successful. Many accommodations for mental health issues are inexpensive and involve workplace flexibility rather than capital expenditures. A study focusing specifically on accommodations for mental illness reported that 90% of reasonable accommodations cost less than $90 (MacDonald-Wilson, Rogers, Massaro, Lyass, & Crean, 2002).

Table 6-1 provides a list of common functional issues experienced by individuals with psychiatric disabilities and, for each issue, outlines suggestions for accommodations that could be put in place. It is important to note that this chart is a starting point only. There are other accommodation strategies that may not be listed here, and the strategy used may depend on the type and degree of limitation experienced by the employee. The desirability of each strategy will also vary depending on the employee and employer.

It is important to note that no two people experience a mental health problem in the same way. Abilities and challenges also change over time and, therefore, supports in the workplace need to be tailored to each client and phased in and out as needed. Negotiating job accommodations is a process that evolves over time and involves a number of potential stakeholders, including supervisors, human resource personnel, occupational health providers, and union representatives (Stergiou-Kita et al., 2010). As part of this process, it is important to remember that all employees with a disability are legally entitled to workplace accommodation. The success of this process, however, is dependent upon good communication between all parties involved. Table 6-2 outlines a step-by-step approach to negotiating workplace accommodations, from initiating the discussion to follow-up and evaluation. Note that several steps involve negotiation to develop the most acceptable options, based on input from both the employee and employer.

In the process of negotiating accommodations, occupational therapists may be involved in advocating on behalf of their clients. In some cases, however, it may be more appropriate to foster the client's self-advocacy skills. Kevin, for example, is a client who could be supported in advocating for himself. He has the motivation as well as the cognitive and social abilities to speak with an employer on his own behalf. In their article on advocacy in vocational rehabilitation, Stergiou-Kita and colleagues (2010) suggest that the advocate "should ensure that individuals understand their rights, abilities, strengths, and needs in relation to job demands and know how to share this information in a manner that avoids discrimination and stigmatization" (p. 219). Resources regarding duty to accommodate can be found through the Canadian Human Rights Commission (www.chrc-ccdp.gc.ca) and through the National Alliance on Mental Illness (www.nami.org) in the United States. Regardless of who is advocating, try to focus on competencies and contributions that could be made to the workplace as opposed to limitations of the worker.

One other issue to consider in the process of negotiating accommodations is that of disclosure. Eligibility for workplace accommodations is based upon disclosure of some type of disability (Dalgin & Gilbride, 2003). What, when, where, why, and how to disclose, however, is the subject of much debate (Goldberg, Killeen, & O'Day, 2005). As outlined earlier, the meaning of work for many young adults is linked to the assumption of a socially valued role that can lead to positive outcomes in terms of identity, self-esteem, and social integration. Disclosure of mental illness, on the other hand, may lead to the construction of a stigmatized identity in the workplace and experiences of discrimination from others (Dalgin & Gilbride, 2003; Ralph, 2002). Many individuals choose not to disclose and are able to function quite well at work (Moll and Workplace Project Committee, 2007). Disclosure may become a necessity, however, if workplace accommodations are needed. Some type of disclosure may also be part of the process of job development. The

Table 6-1. Workplace Accommodation Ideas	
Functional Issue	**Accommodation Ideas**
Decreased stamina	• Flexible scheduling; build work tolerance over time • Build in frequent work breaks • Plan self-paced workload with backup to cover as needed • Job coach
Poor concentration	• Reduce distractions in work area • Private office or enclosed space • Music or headset to block out other noises • Reduce interruptions in workspace • Divide large assignments into smaller tasks and goals • Allow for frequent breaks
Difficulty staying organized and meeting deadlines	• Daily to-do lists with checklist to record tasks as they are completed • Calendars to mark meetings and deadlines • Electronic organizers with cues/timers for completion
Memory deficits	• Record meetings with supervisor and/or team • Provide written instructions • Allow additional training time • Develop written or electronic task checklists
Difficulty handling stress and emotions	• Supervisor or mentor to provide regular praise and positive reinforcement • Allow telephone calls during work hours to access employee assistance or counseling • Allow breaks as needed and arrange for a space to go when stressed • Minimize exposure to emotionally charged situations
Difficulty interacting with others	• Arrange for a quiet space to work as needed • Limit challenging social situations whenever possible (e.g., work from home, communicate via email rather than face to face) • Peer mentor at work to assist with social interaction and "reality checking" as needed • Develop a proactive conflict management plan and include key stakeholders in development and implementation of plan
Adapted from the Job Accommodation Network website http://askjan.org/	

Table 6-2. **The Accommodation Process**	
Step 1: Generate dialogue	• Who are the key stakeholders who need to be involved in the process? • What do you want to disclose about the employee's disability? Consider timing and nature of disclosure.
Step 2: Identify work performance requirements	• What are the essential job tasks? • What are the functional abilities of the employee? • What are the gaps between employee ability and job requirements?
Step 3: Evaluate functional ability of employee	• What limitations is the employee experiencing? • How do these limitations affect job performance?
Step 4: Identify accommodation options	• Generate a list of accommodation options for each performance issue. • Ask the employee and employer what he or she thinks will help.
Step 5: Prioritize strategies	• What does the employee feel is most important? • What is feasible within the workplace? • Does it meet standards for respect, integration, participation, and confidentiality?

Step 6: Establish accommodation plan	• Document a plan and ensure employee and employer are in agreement.
	
	• Plan should include:
	  ◦ Identification of the desired accommodation.
	  ◦ A start date and re-evaluation date.
	  ◦ A timeline for implementation.
	  ◦ A plan for communicating with relevant stakeholders (e.g., supervisors and coworkers).

Step 7: Follow-up	• Monitor implementation. • Revisions to the plan will be needed over time. • Some accommodations may be phased out over time, some may need readjustments, and some may be permanent.

nature of disclosure, in terms of content and timing, however, may vary widely. In order to access accommodations, individuals are not required to reveal their diagnosis; they are only required to identify the functional limitations associated with their illness (Moll et al., 2007). As outlined in Kevin's story, disclosure was not something that he thought about in his early days of working. It was not until after several episodes of his illness and finding an employer that he could trust that he shared his personal history with his supervisor. His experience has been positive, however, he recognizes that this is not the case for everyone. Deciding what to say, when to say it, and to whom is something that should be carefully considered in the SE process.

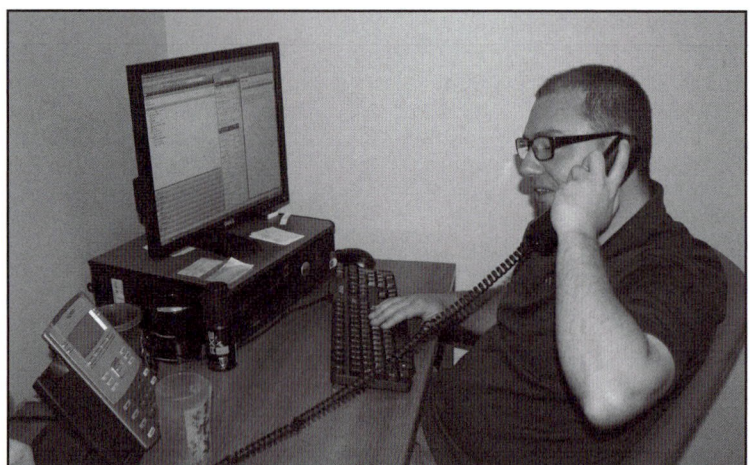

Figure 6-3. Kevin has established work-related skills to meet the demands of the environment and occupation.

Outcomes

The standard outcomes of SE that are reported in the literature include whether the client was able to obtain competitive work, the time to find work, and the duration of employment. Timelines for finding and keeping a job vary, depending upon the client population and nature of the service provided. A study by Cook (1992), for example, compared job tenure of youth versus adults with mental illness and found a significant difference between the two groups. Adults in the study held their independent jobs for an average of 7 months, whereas youth averaged only 3 months at competitive employment. Youth were also significantly more likely than adults to be fired from both placements and independent jobs. A recent study of employment services in New Zealand for young people with mental illness found that 50% to 65% of participants maintained 4 weeks or more of competitive employment, whereas just over one-third of participants accumulated 26 weeks or more of competitive employment (Browne & Waghorn, 2010).

In a SE approach, each work experience is considered to be a new opportunity for learning. If an employee quits or is fired from a position, this should not be viewed as a failure but as a part of the process. The client may have learned something about his or her abilities, needs, and preferences that can be used in finding the next job. Outcomes may therefore relate to the learning that was gained, rather than simply the duration of employment. There is also evidence that with increased work experience, the amount of time in each position typically lengthens, and the time between jobs decreases (Moll et al., 2003). Kevin's story illustrates how "unsuccessful" job experiences can ultimately contribute to increased employment success over time. Clients may need to build his or her skills over time (Figure 6-3).

The desired outcome of SE is competitive work; however, for young people with mental illness, education is an important outcome to track as well. As Kevin's story illustrates, education and employment outcomes are often related; academic upgrading was an important part of his career trajectory. Obtaining academic credentials may enable a client to move beyond an entry-level position to a more meaningful career (Krupa, Woodside, & Pocock, 2010). Successful completion of coursework can also contribute to increased confidence and build skills that are relevant to the work environment (e.g., concentration, attention, time management, and maintaining a regular routine).

In addition to these objective outcomes, it is also important to track the client's perceptions of success. If the clients are satisfied with their job, they are more likely to be successful and stay there for a longer period of time (Rinaldi et al., 2010). One tool that has been developed to measure satisfaction with SE is the Indiana Job Satisfaction Scale. A validation study has been conducted supporting the utility of the tool in vocational rehabilitation with a population of workers with mental health issues (Resnick & Bond, 2001). The Canadian Occupational Performance Measure is another tool that could be used to document a client's perceived satisfaction and performance in relation to his or her work (Law et al., 1998). If a client is not satisfied with his or her job, it is important to gather details regarding the source of the dissatisfaction and proactively address the issues when possible.

Conclusion

An international consensus statement, *Meaningful Lives*, was recently developed to support the rights of young people with a mental illness to pursue employment, education, and training (International First Episode Vocational Recovery Group, 2010). This statement was made in response to the lack of attention paid to functional recovery issues in a system that tends to focus on medical treatment of symptoms, rather than on the evidence regarding the value of education, training, and employment. As outlined in this chapter, work is an important rite of passage in the transition to adulthood and an important part of the recovery process for adolescents and young adults who have experienced mental illness. We can be key service providers and advocates for this population, applying theoretically informed and evidence-based approaches to facilitate employment success.

Review Questions

1. In Kevin's story, what are some of the dimensions of meaning that work had for him during adolescence and young adulthood?

2. What is the current evidence regarding mental illness and its influence on employment?

3. What is the Individual Placement and Support (IPS) model, and how can occupational therapists use this model within his or her own practice?

4. How can occupational therapists measure outcomes of youth and young adults with disabilities and employment?

References

Arbesman, M., & Logsdon, D. W. (2011). Occupational therapy interventions for employment and education for adults with serious mental illness: A systematic review. *American Journal of Occupational Therapy, 65*, 238-246. doi: 10.5014/ ajot.2011.001289

Auerbach, E. S. (2001). The individual placement and support model versus the menu approach to supported employment: Where does occupational therapy fit in? *Occupational Therapy in Mental Health, 17*(2), 1-19. doi: 10.1300/J004v17n02_01

Becker, D. R., & Drake, R. E. (1993). *A working life: The individual placement and support (IPS) program.* Concorde, NH: New Hampshire–Dartmouth Psychiatric Research Centre.

Becker, D. R., Torrey, W. C., Toscano, R., Wyzick, P. F., & Fox, T. S. (1998). Building recovery oriented services: Lessons from implementing individual placement and support (IPS) in community mental health centers. *Psychiatric Rehabilitation Journal, 22*(1), 51-54.

Bell, M. D., & Lysaker, P. H. (1995). Psychiatric symptoms and work performance among persons with mental illness. *Psychiatric Services, 46*(5), 508-510.

Bond, G. R. (2004). Supported employment: Evidence for an evidence-based practice. *Psychiatric Rehabilitation Journal, 27*(4), 345-359. doi: 10.2975/27.2004.345.359

Bond, G. R., Becker, D. R., Drake, R. E., Rapp, C. A., Meisler, N., Lehman, A. F.,...Blyler, C. R. (2001). Implementing supported employment as an evidence-based practice. *Psychiatric Services, 52*(3), 313-322.

Bond, G. R., Drake, R. E., & Becker, D. R. (2008). An update on randomized controlled trials of evidence-based supported employment. *Psychiatric Rehabilitation Journal, 31*(4), 280-290. doi: 10.2975/31.4.2008.280.290

Braveman, B., Robson, M., Velozo, C., Kielhofner, G., Fisher, G., Forsyth, K., & Kerschbaum, J. (2005). *A User's guide to Worker Role Interview, Version 1.0.* Chicago, IL: Model of Human Occupation Clearinghouse, University of Illinois at Chicago.

Brown, C. (2009). Functional assessment and intervention in occupational therapy. *Psychiatric Rehabilitation Journal, 32*(3), 162-170. doi: 10.2975/32.3.2009.162-170

Brown, J. A. (2011). Talking about life after early psychosis: The impact on occupational performance. *Canadian Journal of Occupational Therapy, 78*(3), 156-163. doi:10.2182/cjot.2011.78.3.3

Browne, D. J., & Waghorn, G. (2010). Employment services as an early intervention for young people with mental illness. *Early Intervention in Psychiatry, 4*(4), 327-335. doi:10.1111/j.1751-7893.2010.00188.x

Bryson, G., Bell, M. D., Greig, T., & Kaplan, E. (1999). The Work Behavior Inventory: Prediction of future work success of people with schizophrenia. *Psychiatric Rehabilitation Journal, 20*(4), 113-118.

Bryson, G., Bell, M. D., Lysaker, P., & Zito, W. (1997). The Work Behavior Inventory: A scale for the assessment of work behavior for people with severe mental illness. *Psychiatric Rehabilitation Journal, 20*(4), 47-55.

Bush, P. W., Drake, R. E., Xie, H., McHugo, G. J. & Haslett, W. R. (2009). The long-term impact of employment on mental health service use and costs for persons with severe mental illness. *Psychiatric Services, 60*(8), 1024-1031. doi: 10.1176/appi.ps.60.8.1024

Canadian Institute for Health Information (CIHI). (2005). *Improving the health of young Canadians.* Ottawa, Ontario, Canada.

Carriere, G. (2005). Weekly work hours and health-related behaviours in full-time students. *Health Reports, 16*(4), 11-22. Statistics Canada, Catalogue 82-003.

Case-Smith, J., & O'Brien, J. (2010). *Occupational therapy for children* (6th ed.). London, England: Mosby Elsevier.

Cockburn, L., Kirsh, B., Krupa, T., & Gewurtz, R. (2004). Mental health and mental illness in the workplace: Occupational therapy solutions for complex problems. *Occupational Therapy Now, 6*(5), 7-14.

Cook, J. A. (1992). Job ending among youth and adults with severe mental illness. *Journal of Health Administration, 19*(2), 158-169.

Crowther, R. E., Marshall, M., Bond, G. R., & Huxley, P. (2001). Helping people with severe mental illness to obtain work: Systematic review. *British Medical Journal, 322*(7280), 204-208. doi: 10.1136/bmj.322.7280.204

Dalgin, R. S., & Gilbride, D. (2003). Perspectives of people with psychiatric disabilities on employment disclosure. *Psychiatric Rehabilitation Journal, 26*(3), 306-310. doi: 10.2975/26.2003.306.310

Dickerson, F. B., Stallings, C., Origoni, A., Boronow, J. J., Sullens, A., & Yolken, R. (2008). Predictors of occupational status six months after hospitalization in persons with a recent onset of psychosis. *Psychiatry Research, 160*(3), 278-284. doi:10.1016/j.psychres.2007.07.030

Gioia, D., & Brekke, J. S. (2003). Rehab rounds: Use of the Americans with Disabilities Act (ADA) by young adults with schizophrenia. *Psychiatric Services, 54*(3), 302-304.

Godley, S. H., Passetti, L. L., & White, M. K. (2006). Employment and adolescent alcohol and drug treatment and recovery: An exploratory study. *American Journal on Addictions, 15*(s1), 137-143. doi:10.1080/10550490601006295

Goldberg, S. G., Killeen, M. B., & O'Day, B. (2005). The disclosure conundrum: How people with psychiatric disabilities navigate employment. *Psychology, Public Policy, and Law, 11*(3), 462-500. doi: 10.1037/1076-8971.11.3.463

Goulding, S. M., Chien, V. H. & Compton, M. T. (2010). Prevalence and correlates of school drop-out prior to initial treatment of nonaffective psychosis: Further evidence suggesting a need for supported education. *Schizophrenia Research, 116*(2-3), 228-233. doi:10.1016/j.schres.2009.09.006

Graham, V., Jutla, S., Higginson, D., & Wells, A. (2008). The added value of motivational interviewing within employment assessments. *Journal of Occupational Psychology, Employment, and Disability, 10*(1), 43-52.

Greenberger, E. (1988). Working in teenage America. In J. T. Mortimer & K. M. Borman (Eds.), *Work experience and psychological development through the lifespan* (pp. 21-50). Boulder, CO: Westview.

Griffin, C., Hammis, D., & Geary, T. (2007). *The job developer's handbook: Practical tactics for customized employment.* Baltimore, MD: Brookes.

Gutman, S. A., Kerner, R., Zombek, I., Dulek, J., & Ramsey, C. A. (2009). Supported education for adults with psychiatric disabilities: Effectiveness of an occupational therapy program. *American Journal of Occupational Therapy, 63*(3), 245–254. doi: 10.5014/ajot.63.3.245

Harnois, G., & Gabriel, P. (2002). *Mental health at work: Impact, issues and good practices.* Geneva, Switzerland: World Health Organization. Retrieved from www.who.int/mental_health/media/en/712.pdf

Haslam, J., Pepin, G., Bourbonnais, R., & Grignon, S. (2010). Processes of task performance as measured by the Assessment of Motor and Process Skills (AMPS): A predictor of work-related outcomes for adults with schizophrenia? *Work, 37*(1), 53-64. doi: 10.3233/WOR20101056

Hoff, D., Gandolfo, C., Gold, M., & Jordan, M. (2000). *Demystifying job development: Field-based approaches to job development for people with disabilities.* St. Augustine, FL: Training Resource Network.

Iannelli, S., & Wilding, C. (2007). Health-enhancing effects of engaging in productive occupations: Experiences of young people with mental illness. *Australian Occupational Therapy Journal, 54*(4), 285-293. doi: 10.1111/j.1440-1630.2006.00650.x

International First Episode Recovery Group. (2010). Meaningful lives: Supporting young people with psychosis in education, training and employment: An international consensus statement. *Early Interventions in Psychiatry, 4*(4), 323-326. doi: 10.1111/j.1751-7893.2010.00200.x

Kessler, R. C., Foster, C. L., Saunders, W. B., & Stang, P. E. (1995). Social consequences of psychiatric disorders, I: Educational attainment. *American Journal of Psychiatry, 152*(7), 1026-1031.

Killackey, E. (2010). All in a day's work: opportunities and challenges for vocational interventions in early intervention settings. *Early Intervention in Psychiatry, 4*(4), 267-269. doi:10.1111/j.1751-7893.2010.00202.x

Killackey, E., Jackson, H. J., Gleeson, J., Hickie, I. B., & McGorry, P. D. (2006). Exciting career opportunity beckons! Early intervention and vocational rehabilitation in first-episode psychosis: Employing cautious optimism. *Australian and New Zealand Journal of Psychiatry, 40*(11-12), 951-962. doi: 10.1111/j.1440-1614.2006.01918.x

Killackey, E., Jackson, H. J., & McGorry, P. D. (2008). Vocational intervention in first-episode psychosis: Individual placement and support versus treatment as usual. *British Journal of Psychiatry, 193*(2), 114-120. doi: 10.1192/bjp.bp.107.043109

Kirsh, B. (2000). Work, workers, and workplaces: A qualitative analysis of narratives of mental health consumers. *Journal of Rehabilitation, 66*, 24-30.

Krupa, T., Fossey, E., Anthony, W. A., Brown, C., & Pitts, D. B. (2009). Doing in daily life: How occupational therapy can inform psychiatric rehabilitation practice. *Psychiatric Rehabilitation Journal, 32*(3), 155-161. doi: 10.2975/32.3.2009.155.161

Krupa, T., Woodside, H., & Pocock K. (2010). Activity and social participation in the period following a first episode of psychosis and implications for occupational therapy. *British Journal of Occupational Therapy, 73*(1), 13-20. doi: 10.4276/030802210X12629548272628

Law, M., Baptiste, S., Carswell, A., McColl, M. A., Polatajko, H. J., & Pollock, N. (1998). *Canadian Occupational Performance Measure (COPM)* (3rd ed.). Ottawa, Ontario, Canada: CAOT Publications.

Luecking, R. G. (2008). Emerging employer views of people with disabilities and the future of job development. *Journal of Vocational Rehabilitation, 29*(1), 3-13.

Lysaght, R., Shaw, L., Almas, A., Jogia, A., & Lamour-Trode, S. (2008). Towards improved measures of cognitive and behavioural work demands. *Work, 31*(1), 11-20.

MacDonald-Wilson, K. L., Rogers, E. S., & Anthony, W. A. (2001). Unique issues in assessing work function among individuals with psychiatric disabilities. *Journal of Occupational Rehabilitation, 11*(3), 217-232. doi: 10.1023/A:1013078628514

MacDonald-Wilson, K. L., Rogers, E. S., Massaro, J. M., Lyass, A., & Crean, T. (2002). An investigation of reasonable workplace accommodations for people with psychiatric disabilities: Quantitative findings from a multisite study. *Community Mental Health Journal, 38*(1), 35-49. doi: 10.1023/A:1013955830779

MacDonald-Wilson, K., Rogers, E. S., & Massaro, J. (2003). Identifying relationships between functional limitations, job accommodations and demographic characteristics of persons with psychiatric disabilities. *Journal of Vocational Rehabilitation, 18*(1), 15-24.

McGurk, S. R., Mueser, K. T., Feldman, K., Wolfe, R., & Pascaris, A. (2007). Cognitive training for supported employment: 2-3 year outcomes of a randomized controlled trial. *American Journal of Psychiatry, 164*(3), 437-441. doi: 10.1176/appi.ajp.164.3.437

McMorris, B., & Uggen, C. (2000). Alcohol and employment in the transition to adulthood. *Journal of Health and Social Behavior, 41*(3), 276-294.

Moll, S., Huff, J., & Detwiler, L. (2003). Supported employment: Evidence for a "best practice" model in psychosocial rehabilitation. *Canadian Journal of Occupational Therapy, 70*(5), 298-310.

Moll, S., & Workplace Project Committee. (2007). *When something's wrong: Strategies for the workplace.* Toronto, Canada: Canadian Psychiatric Research Foundation.

Moore-Corner, R. A., Kielhofner, G. & Olson, L. (1998). *A user's manual of work environment impact scale, Version 2.0.* Chicago: Model of Human Occupation Clearinghouse, University of Illinois.

Moos, R. (1994). *Work environment scale manual: Development, applications, research* (3rd ed.). Palo Alto, CA: Consulting Psychologists Press.

Mortimer, J. T. & Staff, J. (2004). Early work as a source of developmental discontinuity during the transition to adulthood. *Development and Psychopathology, 16*(4), 1047-1070. doi: 10.1017/S0954579404040131

Mueser, K. T., Aalto, S., Becker, D. R., Ogden, J., Wolfe, R. S., Schiavo, D.,...Xie, H. (2005). The effectiveness of skills training for improving outcomes in supported employment. *Psychiatric Services, 56*(10), 1254-1260. doi: 10.1176/appi.ps.56.10.1254

Nuechterlein, K., Subotnik, K., Turner, L. R., Ventura, J., Becker, D. R., & Drake, R. E. (2008b). Individual Placement and support for individuals with recent-onset schizophrenia: Integrating supported education and supported employment. *Psychiatric Rehabilitation Journal, 31*(4), 340-348. doi: 10.2975/31.4.2008.340.349

Nuechterlein, K., Subotnik, K., Ventura, J., Gitlin, M., Gretchen-Doorly, G., Green, M.,...Liberman, R. (2008a). A randomized controlled trial of supported employment and education and workplace skills training in recent onset schizophrenia: Notable improvements in work recovery. *Schizophrenia Research, 102*(1-3, supp 2), 1-279. doi: 10.1016/S0920-9964(08)70089-6

Perry, B. M., Taylor, D., & Shaw, S. K. (2007). "You've got to have a positive state of mind": An interpretative phenomenological analysis of hope and first episode psychosis. *Journal of Mental Health, 16*(6), 781-793. doi:10.1080/09638230701496360

Pitts, D. (2011). Work as occupation. In C. Brown & V. Stoffel, (Eds.), *Occupational Therapy in Mental Health: A vision for participation* (pp. 695-710). Philadelphia, PA: F. A. Davis.

Poon, M. Y. C., Siu, A. M. H., & Ming, S. Y. (2010). Outcome analysis of occupational therapy programme for persons with early psychosis. *Work, 37*(1), 65-70. doi: 10.3233/WOR20101057

Porteous, N, & Waghorn, G. (2009). Developing evidence-based supported employment services for young adults receiving public mental health services. *New Zealand Journal of Occupational Therapy, 56*(1), 34-39.

Ralph, R. O. (2002). The dynamics of disclosure: Its impact on recovery and rehabilitation. *Psychiatric Rehabilitation Journal, 26*(2), 165-172. doi: 10.2975/26.2002.165.172

Resnick, S. G., & Bond, G. R. (2001). The Indiana Job Satisfaction Scale: Job satisfaction in vocational rehabilitation for people with severe mental illness. *Psychiatric Rehabilitation Journal, 25*(1), 12-19.

Rinaldi, M., Killackey, E., Smith, J., Shepherd, G., Singh, S. P., & Craig, T. (2010). First episode psychosis and employment: A review. *International Review of Psychiatry, 22*(2), 148-162. doi: 10.3109/09540261003661825

Ryan, M., Marshall, T., Thorburn, B., LeDrew, K., & Hogan, K. (2006). Clients perceptions of factors related to finding and maintaining employment. *Schizophrenia Research, 86*(0920-9964), S146, S379.

Sandqvist, J. L., Bjork, M. A., Gullberg, M. T., Henriksson, C. M., & Gerdie, B .U. (2009). Construct validity of the Assessment of Work Performance. *Work, 32*(2), 211-218. doi: 10.3233/WOR-2009-0807

Singh, S. P., Croudace, T., Amin, S., Kwiecinski, R., Medley, L., & Jones, P. B. (2000). Three year outcome of first-episode psychoses in an established community psychiatric service. *British Journal of Psychiatry, 176*, 210-216. doi: 10.1192/bjp.176.3.210

Stergiou-Kita, M., Moll, S., Walsh, A., & Gewurtz, R. (2010). Health professionals, advocacy and return to work: Taking up the challenge. *Work: A Journal of Prevention, Assessment, and Rehabilitation, 37*(2), 217-223. doi: 10.3233/WOR-2010-1073

Swanson, S. J., & Becker, D. R. (2011). *Supported employment: Applying the individual placement and support (IPS) model to help clients compete in the workforce.* Center City, MN: Dartmouth Hazelden.

Tsang, H. W., Chan, A., Wong, A., & Liberman, R. P. (2009). Vocational outcomes of an integrated supported employment program for individuals with persistent and severe mental illness. *Journal of Behavior Therapy and Experimental Psychiatry, 40*(2), 292-305. doi: 10.1016/j.jbtep.2008.12.007

Tsang, H. W., & Pearson, V. (2001). Work-related social skills training for people with schizophrenia in Hong Kong. *Schizophrenia Bulletin, 27*(1), 139-148.

Vauth, R., Corrigan, P. W., Clauss, M., Dietl, M., Dreher-Rudolph, M., Stieglitz, R. D., & Vater, R. (2005). Cognitive strategies versus self-management skills as adjunct to vocational rehabilitation. *Schizophrenia Bulletin, 31*(1), 55-66. doi: 10.1093/schbul/sbi013

Woodside, H, & Krupa, T. (2010). Work and financial stability in late-onset first-episode psychosis. *Early Intervention Pyschiatry, 4*(4), 314-318. doi: 10.1111/j.1751-7893.2010.00189.x

Woodside, H., Krupa, T., & Pocock, K. (2007). Early psychosis, activity performance and social participation: A conceptual model to guide rehabilitation and recovery. *Psychiatric Rehabilitation Journal, 32*(2), 125-130. doi: 10.2975/31.2.2007.125.130

7

Socialization and Leisure Pursuits for Youth Living With Obesity as the Result of a Complex Health Condition

Mary Forhan, PhD, OT Reg (Ont) and Grace Herron

This chapter provides the reader with the opportunity to explore issues associated with socialization and leisure that are important for an occupational therapist to consider when working with youth during the transition to adulthood. The primary purpose of this chapter is to illustrate ways in which occupational therapists can assess and intervene in the area of socialization and leisure in an outpatient, community-based setting. The secondary purpose of this chapter is to illustrate ways in which occupational therapists can support individuals living with obesity when weight loss is not the primary goal.

Grace's Story

I have struggled with my weight for my entire life. Due to a craniopharyngioma, a reoccurring and benign type of brain tumor located on my pituitary gland, my growth was stunted and my appetite was insatiable. I had my first surgery at the age of 11, during which the tumor was removed. A reoccurrence of the tumor occurred when I was 14 and 19 years old, resulting in more surgery. After each surgical intervention, my weight increased significantly due to the inability of my brain to regulate my hunger and fullness signals. I was always hungry and had very little energy to exercise. At the age of 18, I underwent gastric surgery to decrease the size of my stomach in an effort to control my appetite. The surgery went well, but now I need to be very careful about the foods I eat so that I do not cause damage to my stomach and so that I can control my weight.

Throughout my life, I believe that my weight has had a significant impact on my social life. Changing schools from elementary to secondary school was rough for me because I was growing apart from my elementary school friends, and I had not found anyone else to whom I could relate. I have always been extremely self-conscious about my weight, and because of this, I am hesitant

Stewart, D. (Ed.)
Transitions to Adulthood for Youth With Disabilities
Through an Occupational Therapy Lens (pp. 123-134).
© 2013 SLACK Incorporated

to meet new people. This may be because I have been teased by kids and adults in the past about being overweight. It bothers me that people assume I am overweight because I am lazy and all I do is eat junk food, not because I have a medical condition. But people need to get to know me in order to find this out. I feel lucky to have met someone when I was 16 years old who understands me and what I am going through. She is my best friend, and I can go to her when I am feeling upset, angry, or frustrated and when I want to relax and have some fun. I attended a support group at a children's hospital where there were other kids like me who struggled with their weight. We had a lot of fun together, and it was nice to know I was not alone in my experiences. When I turned 18 years old, however, the group was no longer available to me because I had moved into the adult health care system. No such group existed for young adults with obesity. I also have an extremely supportive family who are willing to help me in any way that they can. Some of them also have challenges with their weight, so we often do active things together to try and stay healthy.

One of the things that most upsets me about my weight is that it often keeps me from doing things that other people my age can do easily, such as running and other sports. I often feel like an older person trapped in a young person's body. I have never really known what it is like to be fit and active. I am on medication for high blood pressure and one of the medication side effects is fatigue, so I have even less energy to do the things I want to do, including being physically active. I often sit back and watch other people doing things that I would love to join in on but do not because I don't have the energy and because I am so self-conscious of my weight and appearance. I would rather hang out with family than friends, because my family members are less judgemental. I recently started university and am starting to make new friends who share similar career goals. Most of the year I live away from home while attending university. I live at home with my family during the summer months or when I need treatment to keep the tumor under control. I have a great relationship with my mother, but sometimes we argue about my weight and exercise. I don't like that my weight is such a public matter, and I would prefer to have an adult relationship with her, focused on friendship and support, not on managing my health condition.

Through an Occupational Therapy Lens

Occupation, Spirituality, and Development

Obesity is associated with health concerns, including hypertension and fatigue, both of which Grace has experienced. The physical health consequences associated with weight are well documented in the literature and are often acknowledged and treated within the medical system (Lau et al., 2007). Less recognized and understood are the psychosocial consequences associated with childhood and adolescent obesity. Weight bias and stigma are associated with bullying behaviors exhibited by children, adolescents, and adults (Craig, Sue, Murphy, & Bauer, 2010). The impact of bullying on children and adolescents impairs self-esteem and self-efficacy. This often results in a decreased sense of self and self-worth and an increase in social isolation (Craig et al., 2010). The actions of well-intended adults and professionals who focus on the negative aspects of a person's weight or force health behaviors, such as exercise or healthy eating, can actually be perceived as bullying for the purpose of shaming someone into action (Puhl & Latner, 2007).

Children and adolescents who are in treatment for obesity are required to practice eating habits that may not fit with the habits of typical children and adolescents, including portion control, timing of meals, and types of food. When foods in a restricted diet are not readily available in schools, shopping malls, and entertainment facilities (i.e., movie theaters or recreation centers), persons in treatment for obesity must bring food with them wherever they go. They are also restricted in their participation in social activities, such as dining out or eating at other people's homes.

Obesity has an impact on the variety of leisure activities available to children and youth, as a result of both the physical consequences of obesity and barriers in the built and social

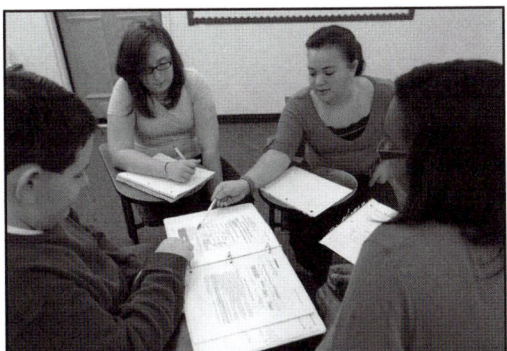

Figure 7-1. All adolescents want to participate in social activities with their peers. (Reprinted with permission from the Rudd Center for Food Policy and Obesity.)

environment. Participation in leisure activities provides important opportunities to develop skills, competencies, and networks of support that are required for the transition to adulthood (Figure 7-1). Children and youth with obesity experience activity restrictions that lead to more passive and socially isolated activities early on in their development. There is, consequently, a risk for adolescents with obesity to transition to adulthood with a smaller network of support and reduced opportunities for developing adult skills and competencies. In fact, it appears that children and adolescents with obesity often have leisure patterns that resemble those of older adults with more time spent on passive activities, done on their own or with one or two other people (Allender, Cowburn, & Foster, 2006; Janssen, Katzmarzyk, Boyce, King, & Pickett, 2004).

Grace has described a desire to be involved in more active leisure activities and to expand her social network. Occupational therapists view participation in leisure activities for adolescents as opportunities to develop skills and competencies and acquire resources and social support networks. Occupational therapists value participation and promote the inclusion of all persons in leisure occupations. The values and beliefs about body weight in North America indicate that an obese body falls outside the norm. It is viewed as deviant and, therefore, not as functional or valuable as that of a body classified as a normal weight (Latner, Stunkard, & Wilson, 2005; Murray, 2007). There are widespread beliefs that obesity is the sole responsibility of the individual and challenges to weight management represent character flaws and negative personality traits. Society, including health professionals and educators, often view persons with obesity as being lazy, less competent, unmotivated, and lacking self-control. Such beliefs create unwelcoming environments for adolescents with obesity who want to participate in leisure activities. There might be physical barriers that limit access to spaces or social barriers, such as the failure to inform or include persons with obesity in leisure opportunities.

Individuals with obesity are often encouraged to focus on reducing their body weight prior to exploring other goals, such as developing a social network, participating in recreational activities, or seeking intimate relationships through activities such as dating. Leisure occupations, including the development of interpersonal relationships, are a primary focus for adolescents and young adults and are highly valued by society. Leisure activities provide opportunities to meet other people, try new things, and find a match between one's abilities, aptitudes, and interests (Figure 7-2). Restricted opportunities in the area of leisure during this transitional stage can have serious repercussions for the development of one's sense of self and the establishment of occupational balance in adulthood (Passmore, 1998).

Understanding the importance of leisure activities and interpersonal relationships for young adults guides the occupational therapist to fully explore these areas with Grace, rather than focusing on past and present medical concerns. Although obesity is a serious health condition, there are

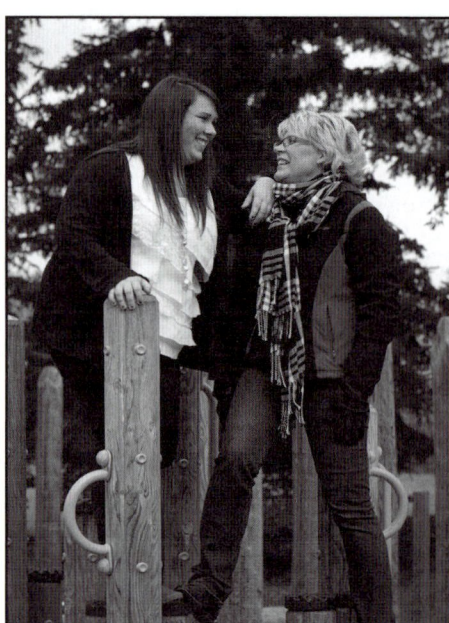

Figure 7-2. Leisure activities provide opportunities for young adults to meet other people and expand occupational interests. (Reprinted with permission from the Canadian Obesity Network.)

other professionals working with Grace to provide knowledge and interventions for her condition. The occupational therapist offers a unique perspective of Grace's experience with obesity and the consequences that weight has had on her daily occupations, especially leisure.

The first interview with Grace took place in an office at the obesity treatment program. The occupational therapist was a consultant contacted from an adult chronic disease management program. It was important for the occupational therapist to reflect on her values and beliefs about obesity prior to meeting the client and to remain client-centered throughout the interview. The purpose of the initial interview was to listen to what Grace had to share about her experience living with obesity and to identify occupational performance issues that are meaningful to her. The Canadian Occupational Performance Measure ([COPM] Law et al., 1998) was used to keep the interview occupation focused and to identify specific occupational performance issues measured in terms of importance, performance, and interest. The results of the COPM are summarized in Table 7-1.

It is clear from the results of the COPM that Grace would like to identify more options for things to do outside of school and family activities, she would like to feel more confident doing these activities, and she would like to have more people involved in her social network of support. In summary, areas that require further assessment are focused on quality, quantity, and confidence in leisure activities.

Person-Environment-Occupation Analysis and Theoretical Approaches

Through further exploration of the occupational performance issues that Grace identified in the COPM, the occupational therapist learns more about person, environment, and occupation (PEO) elements.

Table 7-1. Summary of Canadian Occupational Performance Measure Results			
Occupational Performance Issue	**Importance**	**Performance**	**Interest**
To have more options of things to do in my spare time	7	3	8
To interact with others outside of my family	10	2	10
To build a broader social network	9	4	9

Person

Grace is a motivated young woman who is currently enrolled as a full-time student, participating in courses and working toward a bachelor's degree. Grace has experienced a number of health problems associated with a reoccurring brain tumor. She has experienced a significant weight gain resulting in a body weight classified as obese. She also has hypertension, which is controlled by medications that cause daytime fatigue. Grace has demonstrated the ability to develop and maintain a close, long-term relationship with one peer. She feels most confident with family members and peers in a clinical setting who share similar experiences related to obesity. Grace is interested in expanding her network of friends and would like to try new things. Grace has reported limited confidence in meeting new people due to past social experiences and her thoughts and beliefs about her body size and how she is perceived by others.

Environment

Social interaction and involvement in leisure activities as a young woman is framed by a number of socially ascribed norms and values, including body size. Weight bias and stigma that are demonstrated in the built and social environments, in which most activities take place, are important to consider. Barriers in the built environment include seating that does not support a body weight beyond 250 lbs (115 kg) and seating that is fixed and therefore limits space between seats and tables. Other barriers in the built environment are turnstiles in places such as public transit or theaters and seatbelts on airplanes and motor vehicles that do not extend to adequately support a larger than typical body size. Barriers in the social environment include negative attitudes and beliefs about persons with obesity that result in discriminatory actions, which limit educational, employment, and social opportunities. Weight bias can also result in stereotypes that persons with obesity are less intelligent, leading to lower expectations of adolescents as they transition to adulthood.

Occupation

Social interaction and participation in leisure activities often require time outside of school, money to participate, transportation, and access to various types of activities. Grace lives in an urban area, drives her own car, and has some money available for discretionary use. The developmental expectations of leisure occupations for a young female adult would include a balance of active and passive pursuits and also a balance of individual and social activities. These societal expectations of leisure fit with Grace's own beliefs and expectations. There is also an expectation that a young adult will have had prior leisure experiences upon which to build.

An analysis of PEO reveals that there is a good fit between the environment and occupation in terms of access to leisure activities from a transportation, financial, and resources perspective. There is a poor fit between the social environment, fraught with weight bias and discrimination, and the occupational demands of social interactions.

There is a good person-occupation fit between Grace's motivation and the demands of social interaction and expansion of leisure activities. There is, however, a poor fit between the social demands of leisure occupations and Grace's lack of confidence due to her limited experience with leisure activities and socializing outside of a clinical and family environment.

Based on the analysis of the fit between PEO, the occupational therapist will use both socio-cultural and psychoemotional theoretical approaches to assessment and intervention. These two approaches fit with the identified areas of poor fit between person and social environment (socio-cultural approach) and between personal confidence and occupational demands of social leisure pursuits (psychoemotional approach). The specific conceptual line of inquiry will focus on social networks of support, peer relationships, leisure sense of self, and self-efficacy.

Assessment

In order to recommend the best interventions for Grace, the occupational therapist needs a better understanding of Grace's past and present leisure experiences and current interests. This will guide the development of a list of potential activities and help to identify any barriers or facilitators to Grace's participation in these activities. The occupational therapist could gather this information in an interview by simply asking Grace to recall what leisure activities she used to do, what she currently does, and what she would like to do. Alternatively, using a standard or organized method to collect this information will provide an opportunity to measure changes in Grace's leisure profile after occupational therapy intervention. There are comprehensive leisure assessments available for purchase, which can be useful in identifying specific types of leisure activities a client is interested in and assessing the overall importance of leisure in his or her life (Ragheb & Beard, 1993).

Grace has clearly articulated that she values leisure activities and is requesting an expansion of the types and quality of her leisure participation. Therefore, using a standardized leisure assessment battery with Grace was not necessary or efficient. A modified leisure exploration assessment was conducted with Grace instead, using a leisure inventory table modified after a leisure interest inventory ([Idyll Arbor Leisure Battery] Ragheb & Beard, 1993). The inventory was modified for use with young adults at an obesity treatment program with content that represents a range of current leisure activities, including the use of social media and other technology. The occupational therapist worked through the list of activities on the inventory with Grace during a scheduled office visit. This activity can also be done at home by the client and sent ahead to the therapist to review prior to a scheduled visit. This inventory can also be completed by clients in a group setting, such as an occupational therapist-facilitated leisure interest group. An example of the leisure inventory completed by Grace is found in Table 7-2.

The third occupational performance issue identified by Grace is that of expanding her social network of support. A social network is composed of all of the relationships a person has in his or her life. The purpose and process of each relationship may vary, with some relationships having a clear reciprocal nature of giving and receiving, while others may consist of only giving or receiving. Some relationships are stable while others are ever changing. During the transition from adolescence to adulthood, it is natural for peer and family relationships to evolve as a result of developmental milestones and changes in needs. The health care system demands a change in a young adult's relationship with his or her health care providers by forcing a move to an adult system of care. This is driven by funding models and by the training of health professionals who are often required to delineate expertise and knowledge in either pediatric or adult care.

In order to identify gaps in Grace's current social network, we will need to assess the content, function, and purpose of the network. This can be done using a social network map, in which Grace will be asked to identify people she interacts with and the nature of each relationship (i.e., friend, family member, professional, or work/school contact). A social network map is a useful tool to use during both the assessment and intervention phases of occupational therapy. A social network map is a nonstandardized assessment tool used for the purpose of identifying and better understanding a client's social resources (Hawe, Webster, & Shiell, 2004; Samuelsson, Thernlund, & Ringstrom, 1996; Tracy & Whittaker, 1990). More specifically, it provides a cursory description of the quality and utilization of identified resources. Knowing that Grace prefers to draw diagrams

Table 7-2. Completed Leisure Interest Inventory for Grace			
Activity	**Have Participated in the Past**	**Currently Participate in**	**Would Like to Participate In**
Volleyball			
Soccer	X		
Tennis			
Bike-riding	X		X
Hiking			X
On-line gaming	X	X	
Singing			X
Going to concerts/plays	X		
Dancing			X
Photography			X
Knitting			
Playing cards		X	
Doing puzzles	X		
Skiing			
Boating			
Cultural (festivals, museums, galleries)	X	X	X
Amusement parks			X
Shopping	X	X	X
Camping			X
Movies	X	X	X
Cooking	X	X	
Reading	X	X	X
Gardening	X		
Volunteer work	X		X

than fill out charts, the occupational therapist asked Grace to draw a diagram of her relationships. Grace chose to be creative in how she illustrated the emotional strength of her relationships by using bold letters. She opted to underline those people in the network with whom she would like to have a stronger connection with and put an asterisk beside those people she would like to spend more time with. This helped to describe the relationships in more detail and provide Grace with a visual of her existing network. An example of a social network map completed in an occupational therapy session with Grace is found in Figure 7-3. The social network map can be completed with clients individually or in a group setting.

The occupational therapist will be guided by a psychoemotional approach when addressing Grace's occupational performance issue of interacting with others. The focus will be on Grace's current level of confidence and self-efficacy, as these were identified by her as contributing factors in this occupational performance issue. Grace's history reveals a lifelong experience of interacting with others in a society that values thinness and has misperceptions about the etiology of obesity. Grace described avoiding new relationships and losing old relationships because of her body weight. Grace attributes her self-esteem to her interactions with others. It will, therefore, be

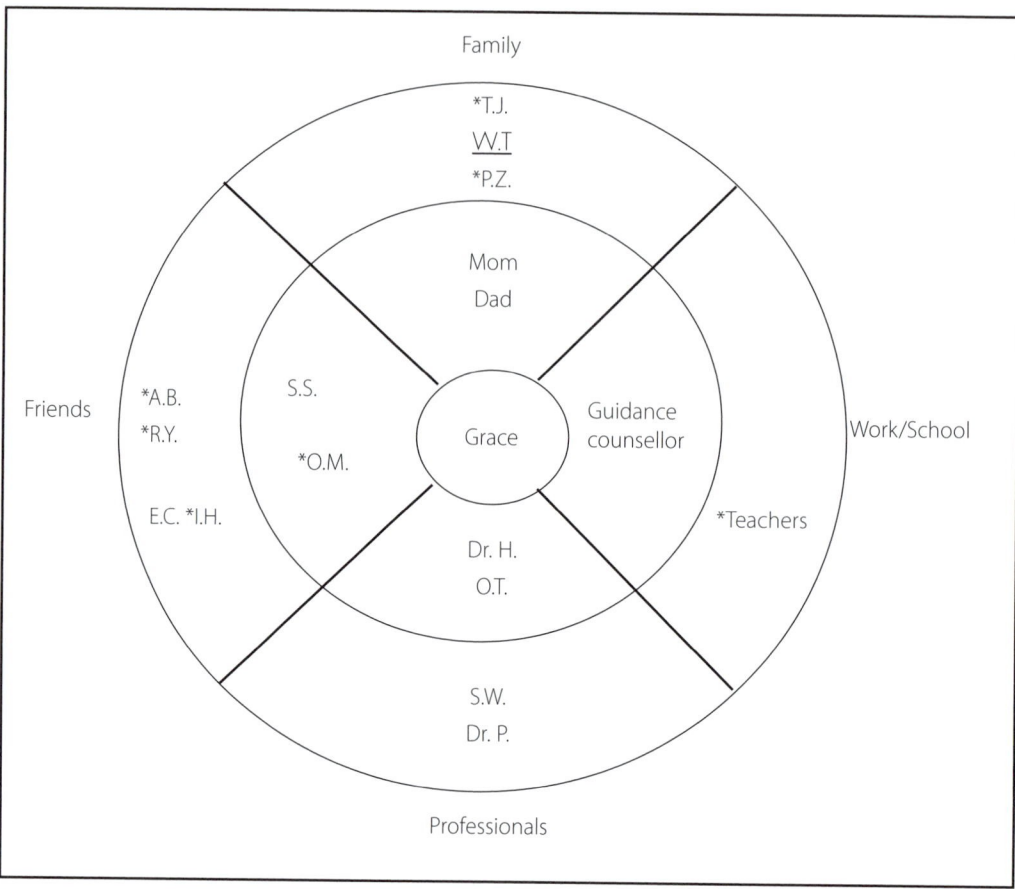

Figure 7-3. Social network map.

important to assess changes in Grace's level of self-esteem over time. A baseline measure of self-esteem will be obtained using the Rosenberg Self-Esteem Scale (Rosenberg, 1989).

Fine Tuning

Based on the assessment results, the psychoemotional and sociocultural approaches are still relevant as the occupational therapist moves into the intervention phase. By viewing Grace's situation through the occupational therapy lens, involvements in structured leisure activities in the community are addressed through a combination of psychoemotional and sociocultural theories.

Intervention

Formal leisure intervention programs for young adults exist in many communities. These programs, however, typically target at-risk youth or individuals in residential or institutional settings. Grace would not meet the criteria to participate in such groups nor would they be the best fit for her. Local community centers and recreational facilities have started to offer leisure programs for young adults with a focus on building self-esteem, expanding social networks, and promoting health and wellness. Activities focus on providing opportunities for physical activity and/or opportunities to try out a variety of new activities in a supportive environment. Although not all programs are explicitly occupation focused, most use leisure activities as a conduit for building networks, increasing capacity and competence, and defining a leisure sense of self. Grace will have access to activities that are matched in terms of age and skill set, providing an opportunity to interact with peers who are also living independently in the community and who share an interest in interacting with others.

The occupational therapist met with Grace at an office in the outpatient rehabilitation department. The first treatment session focused on the information gathered from the leisure interest inventory and was designed to enable Grace to identify resources for exploring the activities she identified an interest in doing. The occupational therapist provided a resource tracking form to help Grace record information about various resources in her home and school community where she could explore leisure interests. The occupational therapist instructed Grace on how to use the recording form and worked with Grace to begin exploring resources using the Internet and key search terms. An example of the completed form is listed as Figure 7-4.

The occupational therapist encouraged Grace to complete the resource tracking form at home and to bring it with her to her next appointment scheduled for later that same week. Grace was asked to identify at least one activity on the list and make a plan to participate in it within 2 weeks. Grace identified the photography classes and theater group as activities she would begin right away. By the end of 2 weeks, Grace had registered for the photography classes and confirmed her attendance at the hometown theater's open house.

Having someone to participate in activities with was a goal for Grace, but she also knew that by asking her close friend or a family member to take photography lessons with her she would not be forced to meet new people. Grace was aware that if she attended classes with someone she already knew, she might only interact with that person and miss opportunities to interact with others. However, Grace expressed feeling anxious about going to the theater open house on her own and opted to bring her friend along. Grace stated that even if her friend also joined the theater company, they would be doing different things as Grace would like to act and her friend would prefer to design sets for the stage. Thus, they would be interacting with different groups of people.

As Grace participated in activities using the resources she identified, she was encouraged to record details important to her about the outcome. Such details could include how she felt prior to, during, and after the activity. During weekly follow-up sessions over the course of 6 weeks, Grace worked with the occupational therapist to identify changes to her social network. This was done by adding initials of individuals who Grace met and interacted with at her formal leisure activities, and also any spontaneous relationships that may have emerged over the weeks.

Grace decided to start a journal to keep track of her feelings and experiences. She stated that since she was making an effort to explore things that were important to her, she would like to document this journey. Grace stated that the purpose of the journal was to have information that she could use to reflect on her feelings, behaviors, and outcomes. She stated that she planned to be constructive in her comments about herself and to try and focus on what she had achieved rather than what she would like to do. The occupational therapist supported Grace in this activity by including reflective exercises in their sessions when Grace opted to share sections of her journal. The occupational therapist also worked with Grace to develop the skill of constructive feedback, with a focus on achievements and ability. Writing a journal and reviewing the contents with a mentor, such as an occupational therapist, is effective for personal development, specifically raising self-awareness and identifying personal strengths and abilities (Langer, 2009; Young, 2010). Reflective writing can also be used as a method for the evaluation of outcomes.

Outcomes of Interest

The evaluation of outcomes took place at each session through the review of the resource tracking form. At each visit, the occupational therapist would review the progress made with Grace and discuss the outcomes identified. In sessions 3 to 4 (out of 10), Grace came to the sessions with the outcome left blank. During a focused discussion with the occupational therapist about her

Resource Name	Description	Contact Information	Date Contacted	Outcome
Young Adult Theatre Company	• Fall/Winter and Spring/Summer sessions for youth ages 17 to 25 • Opportunities for writing scripts, creating set designs, sewing costumes, hair and make-up design, and acting	Hometowntheatregroup@home.com		• Registered to attend the open house with my friend • Plan to talk to someone about acting
Out About Town Social Program for Young Adults	• Session starting in early May designed for college and university students who are home for the summer and want to explore social opportunities in their community • Activities include dinner clubs, book clubs with authors, hiking, art and music tours, picnics, and overnight trips	Allabouttown@home.com		
Recreation and Parks Department of "My City"	• Art classes, salsa dancing, yoga, fun fit classes, photography, and community gardening program with seniors			• Registered for photography classes • Attending once a week on my own • Have arranged photography shoots with a classmate on the weekend at the local park
"My University"	Clubs and activities offered by: • Student union • Recreation/sports complex • University arts and theatre group • Volunteer opportunities throughout campus	 Student union president office (xxx) xxx-xxxx or president@xxxxx.edu.ca contact@rec.ca contact@university-arts.ca contact@volunteeroncampus.ca		

Figure 7-4. Completed resource tracking form.

Table 7-3.					
Summary of Canadian Occupational Performance Measure Results Pre- and Post-Occupational Therapy Interventions					
Occupational Performance Issue	**Importance**	**Performance**		**Interest**	
	Pre	Pre	Post	Pre	Post
To have more options of things to do in my spare time	7	3	8	8	8
To interact with others outside of my family	10	2	6	10	10
To build a broader social network	9	4	7	9	9

experiences since the last session, the occupational therapist worked with Grace to complete this section of the form. This provided an opportunity for Grace to identify outcomes of importance to her, to practice how to document her experiences, and to reflect on them in relation to her occupation-based goals.

The occupation-based issues most important to Grace fall in the area of leisure and include having more options of things to do in her spare time, feeling more confident socializing with others outside of her family, and having a broader social network. The COPM was readministered to Grace in the second to last occupational therapy session. This was done to measure changes in performance and satisfaction for the occupational performance issues identified at the start of occupational therapy with Grace. This will provide Grace and the occupational therapist with perspective on the effectiveness of the occupational therapy intervention in (a) raising awareness about leisure interests, (b) generating and utilizing resources to pursue these interests, (c) building Grace's confidence in her ability to socialize with others outside of her family, and (d) raising awareness about her social network and ways in which to make changes to it. The results of the COPM that were administered post-intervention are found in Table 7-3. The results indicate that Grace perceives her performance in all areas to have improved, however, she would like to improve further in the area of confidence and broadening her social network. These are areas in which we can expect Grace to continue to work on outside of formal occupational therapy sessions. The interventions initiated during occupational therapy were designed to provide Grace with the knowledge and skills required to continue to strengthen occupational performance in leisure after discharge from formal occupational therapy services.

Additional Settings in Which to Work With Young Adults Who Have Obesity

This chapter focused on working with a client whose primary goals focused on socialization in the context of the occupations associated with leisure. The occupational therapist could also work with clients who have obesity with a primary goal of weight loss. The focus then would be on leisure activities that promote physical activity and support eating behaviors required to reduce energy intake or meet the mechanical requirements post-surgery that alter the gastrointestinal tract. In these situations the occupational therapist would review the goals and interests of the client with additional attention to the physical demands required for weight loss activities and the physical ability of the client. The role of the occupational therapist would be to find the best fit between the physical leisure activities and required eating behaviors with those of the client's ability, resources, and values. The occupational therapist would also need to consider how these required activities are integrated or added to the existing occupations the client needs or wants to do. The setting could be a presurgical outpatient clinic, an inpatient post-surgical unit, a primary health care center, or a specialized bariatric program.

The role of occupational therapy working with clients in the area of obesity prevention, treatment, and management is emerging. Occupational therapists have the clinical reasoning and skills to work with this population; however, education, training, and updating of curriculum is needed to provide opportunities to demonstrate the translation of the art and science of occupational therapy to the area of obesity.

Review Questions

1. What are some of the consequences or barriers that Grace experienced due to her health condition?

2. Compare Grace's prior experiences with leisure activities to the developmental expectations of a young adult female. How are they different/similar? What impact might this have on Grace's overall development and well-being?

3. Can you describe the occupational therapy view and role in the importance of leisure activities?

4. What theoretical approaches did the occupational therapist use for assessment and intervention?

5. What resources or assessment tools did the occupational therapist use with Grace?

References

Allender, S., Cowburn, G., & Foster, C. (2006). Understanding participation in sport and physical activity among children and adults: A review of qualitative studies. *Health Education and Research, 21*(6), 826-835. doi: 10.1093/her/cyl063

Craig, W. M., Sue, J., Murphy, A., & Bauer, J. (2010). Understanding and addressing obesity and victimization in youth. *Obesity Management, 6*, 12-16. doi: 10.1089/owm.2010.0103

Hawe, P., Webster, C., & Shiell, A. (2004). A glossary of terms for navigating the field of social network analysis. *Journal of Epidemiology and Community Health, 58*, 971-975. doi:10.1136/jech.2003.014530

Janssen, I., Katzmarzyk, P. T., Boyce, W. F., King, M. A., & Pickett, W. (2004). Overweight and obesity in Canadian adolescents and their association with dietary habits and physical activity patterns. *Journal of Adolescent Health, 35*(5), 360-367. doi: 10.1016/j.jadohealth.2003.11.095

Kjonniksen, L., Torsheim, T., & Wold, B. (2008). Tracking of leisure-time physical activity during adolescence and young adulthood: A 10-year longitudinal study. *International Journal of Behavioral Nutrition and Physical Activity, 5*, 69. doi: http://www.ijbnpa.org/licenses/by2.0

Langer, A. M. (2009). Measuring self-esteem through reflective writing: Essential factors in workplace development for inner-city adults. *Reflective Practice, 10*(1), 45-48. doi: 10.1080/14623940802652755

Latner, J. D., Stunkard, A. J., & Wilson, G. T. (2005). Stigmatized students: Age, sex and ethnicity effects in the stigmatization of obesity. *Obesity Research, 13*(7), 1226-1231. doi: 10.1038/oby.2005.145

Lau, D., Douketis, J., Morrison, K., Hramiak, I., Sharma, A. M., & Ur, E. (2007). 2006 Canadian clinical practice guidelines on the management and prevention of obesity in adults and children. *Canadian Medical Association Journal, 176*, 1-118. doi: 10.1503/cmaj.061409

Law, M., Baptiste, S., Carswell, A., McColl, A., Polatajko, H .J., & Pollock, N. (1998). *The Canadian Occupational Performance Measure (COPM)* (3rd ed.). Ottawa, Ontario, Canada: CAOT Publications ACE.

Murray, S. (2007). Corporeal knowledges and deviant bodies: Perceiving the fat body. *Social Semiotics, 17*(3), 361-373. doi: 10.1080/10350330701448694

Passmore, A. (1998). Does leisure support and underpin adolescents' developing worker role? *Journal of Occupational Science, 5*(3), 161-165.

Puhl, R. M., & Latner, J. D. (2007). Stigma, obesity and the health of the Nation's children. *Psychological Bulletin, 133*(4), 557-580. doi:10.1037/0033-2909.133.4.557

Ragheb, M. G., & Beard, J. G. (1993). *Idyll Arbor Leisure Battery.* Enumclaw, WA: Idyll Arbor Inc.

Rosenberg, M. (1989). *Society and the adolescent self-image.* (Rev. ed.). Middletown, CT: Wesleyan University Press.

Samuelsson, M., Thernlund, G., & Ringstrom, J. (1996). Using the five field map to describe the social network of children: A methodological study. *International Journal of Behavioural Development, 19*, 327. doi: 10.1177/016502549601900206

Tracy, E. M., & Whittaker, J. K. (1990). The social network map: Assessing social support in clinical practice. *Families in Society, 71*(8), 461-470.

Young, K. L. (2010). Learning through reflective writing: A teaching strategy. *Evidence Based Library and Information Practice, 5*(4), 96-98. doi: http://ejournals.library.ualberta.ca/index.php/EBLIP/article/view/9146

Future Directions in Practice and Research

Our Own Transitions

Debra Stewart, MSc, OT Reg (Ont)

> Jenny is 5 years old and lives with her parents and older brother. Her parents noticed that her verbal skills were not progressing as a preschooler and that she did not play with other children, so they took her to see a developmental pediatrician. A diagnosis of autism spectrum disorder (ASD) was made, and her parents found a preschool program that provided extra supports for children with autism. They have decided to enroll her in kindergarten in the public education system this coming fall, as they have heard there is an autism team within the school system.

How can we as occupational therapists use and build upon the current evidence about transitions to adulthood for youth with disabilities in the next 15 years so Jenny will be able to achieve her desired outcomes as a young adult? What needs to happen within systems and services between now and then to meet Jenny's needs for a smooth, successful transition to adult life? The evidence presented in this book provides a starting point to identify what is already known (and can be built upon) and what is not known. This information should give occupational therapists and other professionals working with children and youth with disabilities some directions for the future.

What Do We Know?

Every transition journey is unique and clinicians, therefore, need to address each person's journey in an individualized and client-centered manner. Although each individual is unique, evidence indicates that many of the issues and challenges facing youth with any type of disability are similar. For example, all youth with disabilities have poorer adult outcomes than those without disabilities in the domains of employment, post-secondary education, living arrangements, and

Stewart, D. (Ed.)
Transitions to Adulthood for Youth With Disabilities Through an Occupational Therapy Lens (pp. 135-152).
© 2013 SLACK Incorporated

socialization (Wagner, Newman, Cameto, Levine, & Garza, 2006). They also face fewer opportunities and more challenges to full participation than their nondisabled peers. It is now known that experiences and opportunities during childhood and adolescence can have positive impacts on future adult occupations (Gorter, Stewart, & Woodbury-Smith, 2011). Occupational therapists need to build on this evidence to identify meaningful experiences and opportunities for Jenny throughout childhood and adolescence.

Various factors within the person and the environment influence the transition process. Recent evidence is showing how these factors interact with each other, and the fit between person and environment (and occupation from an occupational therapist's view) influences the perception of these factors. If there is a good fit between person and environment (and occupation), then the factors are perceived to be supportive (e.g., parents who provide transportation for their youth to participate in social pursuits with friends). When there is a poor fit between person, environment, and occupation (PEO), the factor of interest is perceived to be a barrier or a hindrance to the transition process (e.g., when school personnel's low expectations of a youth prevent him or her from participating in a co-op program). Occupational therapists have a strong understanding of PEO fit and how to improve this fit through modifying the environment or occupation to enable participation. We can, therefore, contribute to knowledge development in this area.

Transition services are being implemented within education, health care, developmental, social, mental health, and other systems. Although research about the effectiveness of transition services is still very limited, there is some preliminary evidence emerging that supports different types of programs. For example, in the health care literature, programs that focus on self-management (Mahmood, Dicianno, & Bellin, 2011), parent support groups (Kingsnorth, Gall, Beayni, & Rigby, 2011) and socioecological elements of the transition process (Schwartz, Tuchman, Hobbie, & Ginsberg, 2011) are showing promising results.

Legislation is starting to have an impact in positive ways on the post-school outcomes of youth with disabilities (Luecking & Wittenburg, 2009). However, recent research suggests that legislation needs to address all aspects of adult transitions (Committee on Disability in America, 2007; Learning Disabilities Association of Canada ([LDAC)], 2007) to achieve positive outcomes for all youth.

What Do Not We Know Yet?
(What Are Our Knowledge Gaps?)

The various processes of the dynamic interactions of the PEO factors involved in transitions to adulthood are not yet well understood. Research that is multifactorial and multidimensional in nature is needed to understand dynamic, developmental processes. Recent developmental theories that address these interactions and focus on positive developmental trajectories should guide us (Halfon & Hochstein, 2002; Hawkins et al., 2011). A lifecourse approach to transition and disability (Leiter & Waugh, 2009; Priestly, 2001) has some good theoretical evidence to support its use in research and clinical practice, and it is something about which we need to learn more.

Although there is some emerging evidence about the effectiveness of specific services within a system, there is very little evidence about services and supports that address transitions as part of the holistic lifecourse of an individual with disabilities. It is difficult, however, to develop holistic approaches within systems and services without a clear framework, or model, that fosters a collaborative view of all transitions.

Studies have identified the outcomes that matter for youth with disabilities, such as participation, contribution, citizenship, and quality of life (Stewart et al., 2009), but there are very few strong measures for these concepts. The development of participation-level outcome measures for youth with all types of disabilities is needed in order to know what truly makes a difference during transitions to adulthood.

This relatively brief review of evidence is a worthwhile endeavor for practitioners who are working with youth with disabilities. An annual review is strongly recommended as the evidence in this area is building quickly and we are gaining more knowledge every year.

The next question then is how do occupational therapists and other professionals move this evidence into practice at all levels—government, systems and services, communities, and individuals? The remainder of this chapter provides evidence-based recommendations for future directions for systems and services and, specifically, for occupational therapists.

Future Directions for Systems, Services, and Supports

A strategy that has been used in many systems and services to move evidence into practice is the development of practice guidelines (MacDermid, 2008). There has been increased interest in practice guidelines among rehabilitation professionals in the past decade (MacDermid, 2008). The evidence in this book suggests that collaborative guidelines are needed that are useful for more than one discipline or service. Guidelines to support communities to develop a holistic lifecourse approach to transitions to adulthood would appear to make the most sense, given the current evidence. Although this may take more effort on the part of the people working in different systems and services, this is a direction we need to move in if we want youth with all types of disabilities to achieve positive and meaningful adult outcomes.

An example from the local community of Hamilton, Ontario, Canada is presented next to demonstrate how a transition network used current evidence and shared knowledge to develop collaborative community-based guidelines. The network included researchers; educators; service providers from the whole province of Ontario representing different systems; community members, such as employers and recreation leaders; policy analysts; and most importantly, youth with disabilities and his or her family members. The members of this transition network had worked together in research projects and resource development for youth with disabilities over the past 10 years and they were at a stage of wanting to put the evidence into practice. Consensus meetings were held to review the current evidence and identify guidelines. The result of this work was a document that included a generic model for transition to adulthood for youth with disabilities in our province, the—Best Journey to Adult Life (BJA) model—and guidelines for best practice for individuals, communities, services, and governments (Stewart et al., 2009).

The BJA model is represented metaphorically as a series of journeys in hot air balloons. Network participants wanted to acknowledge the multiple transitions that youth and families experience but could not find a graphic model in the current literature that was truly collaborative and lifecourse-oriented. The hot air balloon metaphor acknowledged that an individual experiences a series of transition stages—preparation, the journey itself, and the landing—after which the individual begins to prepare for the next transition. Figure 8-1 provides a visual representation of this model.

Guidelines for best practice were organized into four themes (Stewart, 2009; Stewart et al., 2009). These themes are used in the following sections to frame recommendations for future evidence-based practice in systems and services.

Theme 1: Collaborative Initiatives and Policies for Transitions to Adulthood Are Needed

The evidence is clear that everyone must work together to address the multiple adult transitions of youth with disabilities in a holistic, lifecourse approach (Stewart et al., 2008). Collaboration is needed at many levels. At the macro level of government and policy, separate divisions or ministries are addressing issues of transition to adulthood for youth with disabilities, such as education, health, social, developmental services, housing, transportation, disability supports, and employment. Many government reports, policy briefs, and legislation up until now tend to be focused on one area or domain of transition that is relevant for that government sector (e.g., the Rehabilitation

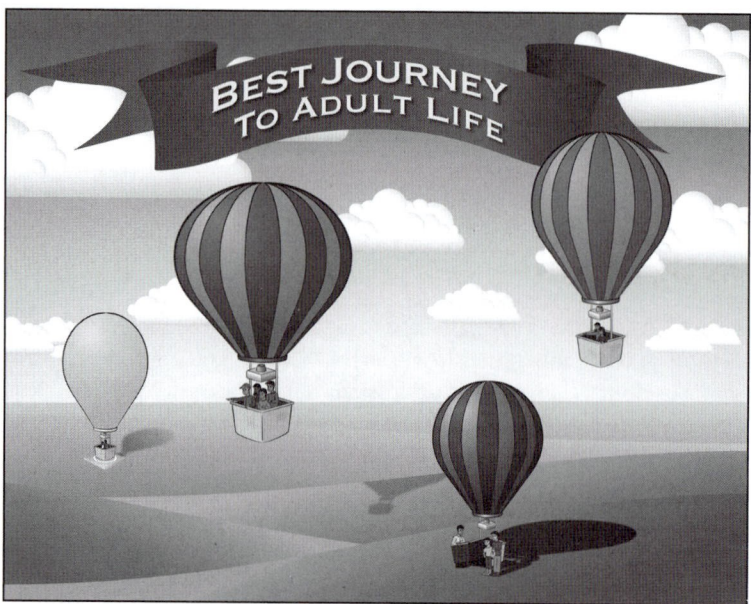

Figure 8-1. Graphic representation of the Best Journey to Adult Life. (Reprinted with permission from Stewart, D., Freeman, M., Law, M., Healy, H., Burke-Gaffney, J., Forhan, M.,...Guenther, S. [2009]. *"The best journey to adult life" for youth with disabilities. An evidence-based model and best practice guidelines for the transition to adulthood for youth with disabilities.* Hamilton, Ontario, Canada: McMaster University. Retrieved October 30, 2011 from http://transitions.canchild.ca/en/OurResearch/bestpractices.asp)

Act focuses more on health care transitions). However, there are some collaborative policy activities that are now focusing on the whole picture of transition. In the United States, the reauthorization of the Individuals with Disabilities Education Act (IDEA) in 2004 as P.L.108-446 expanded the focus of the legislation from just special education to include related service partners and transition plans (Spencer, 2010). In the United Kingdom, the Autism Act (2009) acknowledges the need for many services and systems to work collaboratively toward positive outcomes for adults with autism spectrum disorder (ASD) (McConachie, 2011). The future will hopefully see more legislation that mandates collaborative transition planning and service delivery across all sectors and systems. This direction will promote knowledge development about transitions for all youth.

At the system and services level, most evidence comes from system-specific research and programs (Gorter et al., 2011). While these activities have helped each system and service to identify the needs of the population(s) they serve, they foster a focus on specific components based on system needs rather than looking at the whole person. Efforts are apparent in recent literature to encourage collaboration between systems (Repetto, Gibson, Lubbers, Gritz, & Reiss, 2008) and to improve the coordination between pediatric and adult services and systems (Gorter et al., 2011), but much more is needed if we want to provide seamless service transitions.

At the community level, collaboration is needed between the different agencies and community supports that youth with disabilities can access. Evidence-based recommendations for this level of collaboration include the formation of a community transition network, funding of a community transition coordinator, and adding information about disability-related services and supports to community-based resources and Web sites (Stewart et al., 2008).

Most importantly, more active collaboration is needed between service providers, youth, and families. Any new initiative related to the transition to adulthood should include youth and families at the planning table. Any research in this area should have youth and parents as active members of the research team. This should become expected policy and procedure at all levels. It is through these types of collaborations that knowledge and evidence for the future is built.

TABLE 8-1.
Principles of Community Capacity Building
• Reflect the values of community development.
• Be driven by the community's priorities.
• Take the existing strengths and talents within the community as the starting point for development.
• Be of benefit to the individuals directly involved and to their own wider community.
• Empower people to act on behalf of their community.
• Learn from best practice in other communities.
• Establish and strengthen new and existing networks.
Reprinted with permission from Department for Social Development. (2009). Voluntary and community sector community capacity building. Northern Ireland, UK. Retrieved October 30, 2011 from www.dsdni.gov.uk/vcni-community-capacity-building.pdf.

One of the barriers to collaboration is the lack of a unified framework or model of transition to adulthood that could guide all systems and services to work together. Although this may seem difficult to achieve, a collaborative model would encourage a merging of views about adult transitions and move us all in the same direction (Hamdani, Jetha & Norman, 2011). One recommendation from the evidence presented in this book would be to consider the use of the model of functioning in the International Classification of Functioning, Disability and Health (ICF; see Figure 1-5) (World Health Organization [WHO], 2001). This model can encourage intersectoral discussions about the interactions between person and environment and the different levels of functioning that can be addressed. The ICF model does have the potential to promote collaboration across different systems because of its biopsychosocial perspective (Stewart & Rosenbaum, 2007). However, health care professionals will need to explain the broadened view of health that is imbedded in the ICF to other team members. Professionals who are not part of the health care system may only know the traditional, narrow perspective of the term *health* that was part of the medical model. If everyone's view of health can be expanded to include concepts of activities, participation, and person-environment interactions, then transition teams may be interested in adopting the ICF model to guide service delivery. This would be a positive first step.

Theme 2: Building the Capacity of the Whole Community

The term *capacity* represents a shift away from simple skill development in a particular area of function such as physical skills, academic skills, or vocational skills to address the current and future abilities and assets of each individual. Individual capacity includes knowledge and skills, resources, strengths, and experiences that all contribute to participation in daily life (Stewart et al., 2009).

Capacity is described as the "ways and means needed to do what has to be done" (Department for Social Development [DSD], 2009, p. 3). The term *capacity* can be applied to all individuals within a community, not just youth with disabilities. Individuals may include families, neighbors, employers and employees, agency and service personnel, and other community members. Their knowledge, skills, resources, and experiences can all be used in a positive and strengths-based approach to include everyone in community life. The capacity of a community as a whole can be built by focusing on the resources, partnerships, and opportunities available and accessible for youth with disabilities (DSD, 2009). This is a more inclusive and asset-based approach to community development. Some of the key principles of community-capacity building are listed in Table 8-1. There are many resources available for communities interested in capacity-building workshops. A manual written by Kretzmann and McKnight (1983) still serves as a foundational

TABLE 8-2.
Two Definitions of Health Literacy

United States	"The degree to which individuals have the capacity to obtain, process, and understand basic health information and services needed to make appropriate health decisions" (Ratzan & Parker, 2000, as cited in Nielsen-Bohlman, Panzer, & Kindig 2004, p. 20).
Canada	"The ability to access, understand, evaluate, and communicate information as a way to promote, maintain, and improve health in a variety of settings across the life-course" (Rootman & Gordon-El-Bihbety, 2008, p. 11).

resource for building communities through asset-based development and use of capacity inventories.

When capacity building occurs at multiple levels at the same time, the transition process for youth with disabilities is more likely to be a positive experience with positive outcomes.

Theme 3: Information, Resources, and Services Need to Be Accessible and Available to All

One of the important elements of community capacity building is accessible and useful information and resources about transitions to adulthood and related services and supports (Stewart et al., 2009). Accessibility of information means it is available in user-friendly language and simple technology that is universal and consistent across different systems and services. Information exchange should be in two directions (e.g., youth to service provider and vice versa), as this promotes informed decision making by everyone involved.

The importance of accessible and useful information has gained recognition with increased understanding of the concept of health literacy. At the start of the new millennium, the US Department of Health and Human Services spearheaded a national focus on literacy, after which a report was released by the Institute of Medicine entitled *Health Literacy: A Prescription to End Confusion* (Nielsen-Bohlman, Panzer, & Kindig, 2004). Other countries have also conducted studies and published reports on health literacy (Rootman & Gordon-El-Bihbety, 2008), which provide valuable information for professionals working with youth and families.

Current definitions of the term *health literacy* acknowledge the personal and environmental elements interacting within this complex topic. Definitions from two countries in Table 8-2 show similarities in scope. These definitions of health literacy recognize the importance of information that is accessible and understandable to many different people, at all ages and stages of life. Experts now recognize that people's access to health information and their capacity to use it effectively will improve their sense of empowerment for their own health care (WHO, 1998).

One of the barriers to health literacy is poorly worded information about health issues (Rootman & Gordon-El-Bihbety, 2008). It would seem reasonable that the same applies for information within any system or service context. All professionals need to provide information about the transitions to adulthood for youth with disabilities in useful, understandable, age-appropriate, and context-relevant ways. For youth in particular, information must be presented with a cool factor to which they can relate and understand before they will pay attention.

It seems logical that youth with disabilities would turn to their computers for information about transitioning to adulthood (Figure 8-2). Internet-based information is available to youth in the form of Web sites, chat rooms, Facebook pages, and other forms of social media. One example is "Ability Online" (www.abilityonline.org), which is an internationally renowned online network that provides a safe forum for online peer support for children, youth, and families with chronic

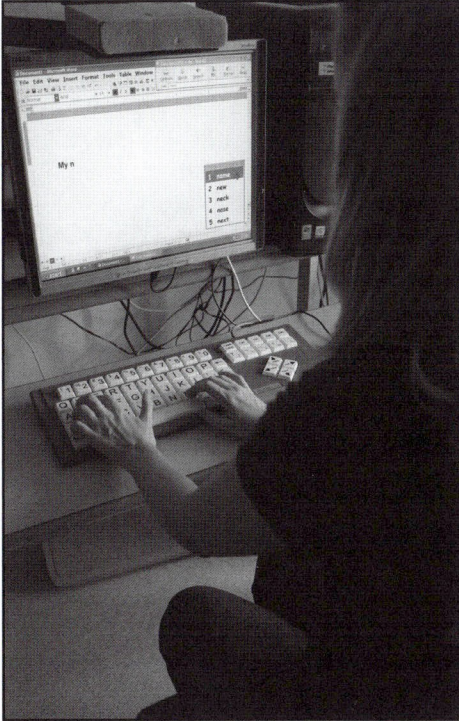

Figure 8-2. Youth use computers to find and share information.

health conditions and special needs. Research has demonstrated the benefits of this online support for youth with chronic medical and physical disabilities (Nicholas et al., 2009; Social Support Research Program, 2005). This type of youth-centered information will hopefully continue to grow in the future.

Theme 4: Education and Research Is Critical for Our Knowledge Development

Knowledge is built through education and research. Education of all service providers is needed about the capacities and needs of youth with disabilities in transition to adulthood. This developmental process should be included in the curricula of professional education programs in health care, education, social services, and any other discipline working with youth.

Any education on the topic of transitions to adulthood and disability should give the audience a vision of a positive future and show the importance of experiential opportunities for children and youth with disabilities as they grow up. All professionals and agency personnel need to know what they can do to promote opportunities for meaningful experiences for youth with disabilities through their childhood, adolescence, and into young adulthood. During childhood, this can be as simple as supporting parents to think about their visions and dreams for their child when they grow up, so they can act early to get the supports needed. As children get older, professionals can collaborate with parents and community members to develop opportunities for adolescents to participate in volunteer and recreational activities in their local community. Health care professionals can support parents and workers to promote a youth's self-determination and ability to direct others by coaching them to wait for the youth to tell them how he or she wants an assisted transfer to be done instead of just automatically doing it.

The evidence is pointing to a knowledge gap in the "adult world" (Stewart et al., 2008). Many youth with disabilities and their families have grown up in their communities, have experienced some level of integration and inclusion, and have received supports when needed. The experiences of youth after transitioning to adulthood are very different, and many feel that the adult world is not ready for these young people (Stewart, Law, Rosenbaum, & Willms, 2001). There appears to be a great need for the education of people in adult communities to increase awareness and understanding of the capacities of young people with disabilities. Greater awareness will then lead to more opportunities in the community for youth with disabilities to participate in recreational, social, educational, volunteer, and paid employment experiences. In a recent Canadian study about the transitional tensions facing youth with disabilities, many of the youth participants indicated that they wanted to be part of this educational process as they felt that "being out there" in the community was the best way to increase awareness and understanding (Stewart et al., 2008).

Research also promotes knowledge and builds capacity. Our best practice guidelines suggest that different types of research are needed at different levels. Although large, rigorous studies provide high-quality information about the effectiveness of services and programs, this type of research takes a long time and is costly. Right now, our services can be evaluated to build evidence of "what works" within practice settings. Any new transition program/service should be evaluated to demonstrate the benefits of the program. This can start with systematic data collection of a new assessment tool or a pre-post evaluation of a new program.

In order to connect research to practice, effective transfer of knowledge is needed. Different models of knowledge transfer and exchange exist in health care and other fields. Some models focus more on ways to change the behaviors of practitioners, while others place emphasis on changing organizational culture and knowledge (Law & Telford, 2008). Whatever model is chosen to guide knowledge transfer and dissemination, there is a need for all stakeholders to be involved to ensure that the different types and levels of information are shared and acted upon (Law & Telford, 2008). It is also important to remember that the needs of clients (youth, families, community members, etc.) are at the center of all knowledge transfer strategies (Ho et al., 2004).

These recommendations for the future are broad in scope at the level of systems, services, communities, and research. The next section will focus specifically on clinical occupational therapy practice and offer recommendations for our own transitions to meet the needs of all youth with disabilities.

Transitions for Occupational Therapists

The authors in this book have provided evidence-based practice strategies that address an individual's occupational performance in different environments. Using a framework such as the McMaster Lens for Occupational Therapists (Salvatori et al., 2006) to guide our reasoning and decision making, occupational therapists can select the ideas in this book that fit best with their setting and the client populations with which they work. Recommendations within the four themes of best practice guidelines described previously are presented within the context of Jenny's scenario to promote the ongoing development of clinical reasoning by connecting research, theory, and practice. The recommendations are focused on our unique clinical reasoning in different practice settings and not about specific assessment or intervention models.

Children with autism can have significant social and communication challenges that impact their participation in daily occupations (Crabtree & DeLany, 2011). Evidence also indicates that youth with autism have poorer adult outcomes than their peers in the all-transition domains (Wagner et al., 2006). The prevalence of autism has increased in the past few decades, and occupational therapists in school systems and pediatric settings typically have many children and adolescents with autism on their caseloads (Crabtree & DeLany, 2011). Resources for service providers have been developed by autism experts (see the Autism Internet Modules at

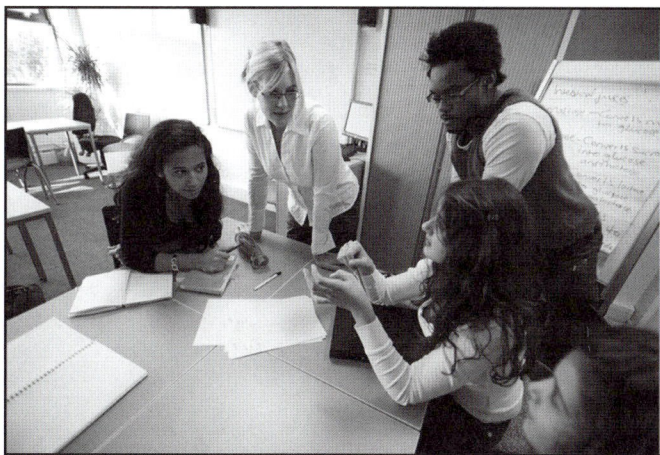

Figure 8-3. In high schools, occupational therapists can meet with students during naturally occuring activities.

www.autisminternetmodules.org) and our national associations are supporting occupational therapy practitioners with useful guidelines and resources (Miller-Kuhaneck, 2004; Tomchek & Case-Smith, 2009). The evidence in this book about transitions to adulthood for youth with disabilities can be added to the clinician's repertoire of clinical reasoning strategies for daily practice.

Collaboration

Occupational therapists who use client- or family-centered approaches when working with children such as Jenny are already collaborating with families to plan and provide services. Client- and family-centered practices that promote collaboration and evidence shows that these approaches to service delivery do make a difference (King, Teplicky, King, & Rosenbaum, 2004; Law, 1998). An important collaborative role of occupational therapists is related to advocacy skills. Therapists who are working with younger children need to help parents develop their own advocacy skills to identify and ask for the supports their children need. Then as children get older, occupational therapists can work with them to develop self-advocacy skills. This can start early by working collaboratively with children and families to encourage a child to begin to advocate for his or her own needs for assistance. For example, occupational therapists can teach basic self-advocacy skills with children in elementary school and their parents to enable them to identify their needs for supports and accommodation during school meetings.

Many occupational therapists are embracing collaboration within education settings (Bazyk & Case-Smith, 2010). The term *school-based collaborative consultation* is defined as "…an interactive team process that focuses student, family, education, and related services partners on enhancing the academic achievement and functional performance of all students in school" (Hanft & Shepherd, 2008, p. 3). Occupational therapists who are part of school-based teams, including specialized autism teams and transition teams, use professional knowledge, skills, and abilities to enable optimal participation and inclusion of students with disabilities. Three key elements of collaborative practice are blended together by therapists working in the school setting: hands-on services in natural settings, team supports, and system supports (Hanft & Shepherd, 2008). In high schools, occupational therapists need to find the best times within a student's naturally occurring routines to provide services and supports (Figure 8-3). This may be in specific classes that embrace a collaborative culture, at lunch time, or when a student is in a resource room or with a peer mentor (Clark, 2008). By working with a student, such as Jenny, in naturally occurring contexts, the occupational therapist is helping to build his or her personal capacities for community participation.

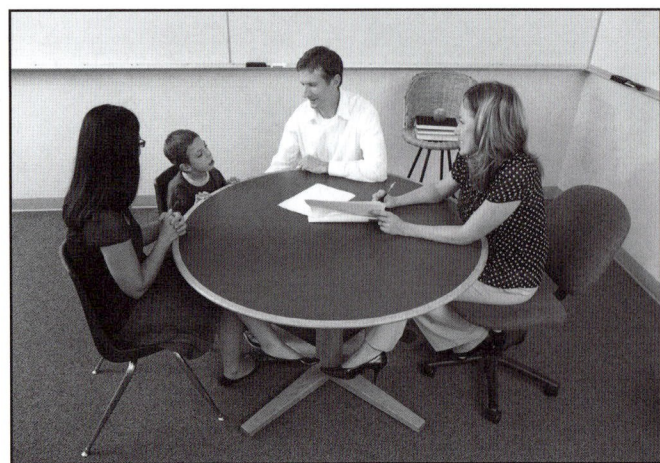

Figure 8-4. Collaboration consultation requires ongoing dialogue and problem solving with teachers, parents, and students.

Evidence is emerging that this service approach contributes to the achievement of goals and skill development, as reported by teachers (Barnes & Turner, 2001; Reid, Chiu, Sinclair, Wehrmann, & Naseer, 2006). Findings from two recent critical reviews of the literature on school-based collaborative consultation suggest that collaborative services can increase teachers' understanding about occupational therapy and also improve their perceptions of how occupational therapists contribute to student achievement (Sayers, 2008; Villeneuve, 2009). Recommendations for occupational therapists using this approach include engaging with educators to clarify expectations and negotiate service delivery approaches; understanding the context of the classroom, school, curriculum, and board policies; and using collaborative consultation with other service models to match intervention strategies with the individual needs of each student (Sayers, 2008; Villeneuve, 2009).

For occupational therapists working with children with disabilities, a collaborative consultation model fits well with a kindergarten environment in the first year of school as we can observe children's participation in the classroom setting and offer a different lens than the teacher's for viewing behaviors and performance (Missiuna et al., 2012). Through ongoing dialogue and problem solving with teachers and parents, strategies can be put in place to enhance participation (Figure 8-4). These strategies can carry over into future grades. Through collaborative activities within the school, the occupational therapist's role will become known by teachers, who can then contact therapists when occupational issues arise instead of waiting until a crisis occurs.

In high school, a collaborative consultation approach can facilitate an inclusive curriculum for all students with special needs (Hines, 2008). Although Jenny may not want to be working directly with the therapist in her classrooms, which is typical of many adolescents, the therapist can be introduced as a related services partner for the whole classroom and observe the interactions to analyze the PEO fit. Then, outside of class time, the therapist can participate in meetings with the principal, teacher, other related services partners, Jenny, and her parents to establish meaningful goals and an inclusive transition plan. The occupational therapist can also support Jenny in continuing to develop her self-advocacy skills within the school system in order to enable her to speak up for her own needs for supports and accommodation. This can be accomplished by encouraging Jenny to contact the occupational therapist herself when she wants to discuss self-advocacy strategies for a particular situation.

Occupational therapists need to collaborate more with each other across different services and systems to better understand the common issues and effective practices for all youth with disabilities. This could start within an institution at departmental meetings to discuss issues related to service transitions. At a community level, therapists could start a transition interest group to share information with each other and develop a practice framework that addresses a lifecourse approach to transition.

Occupational therapists also need to collaborate more with other professionals within the systems providing transition services. Collaborative consultation approaches, as described previously, foster this type of interprofessional connection within the education system. Pediatric therapists need to start connecting with therapists who work with adults with lifelong conditions to learn from each other. The evidence indicates that professionals in adult services do not have the same understanding or motivation to work with young adults with chronic conditions, including those with ASD (Gorter et al., 2011; McConachie, 2011). Youth with ASD are at risk for mental health problems and have ongoing support needs as adults, which are often not being met by adult systems and services (McConachie, 2011). Occupational therapists working in pediatric settings can connect with their counterparts in adult programs to ensure that transitions between occupational therapists are effective in continuing to provide necessary supports and services.

Interprofessional collaboration can be beneficial in sharing ideas and building a more inclusive service community, but it can also be used to advocate for the inclusion of occupational therapists in multidisciplinary transition teams as we have a great deal to offer to these teams. Recent research indicates that occupational therapists are not included in many transition teams (Mankey, 2011). Advocacy efforts can be within an institution—inviting members of a transition team to coffee or lunch to talk about how an occupational therapist could become involved—or at the larger community level by asking to join an existing transition network.

As an aside, occupational therapists who use a collaborative consultation approach could also be offering their knowledge and expertise to a whole school or community regarding transitions to adulthood, and not just for youth with disabilities. Use of the McMaster Lens encourages therapists to focus on occupation first, and to use PEO analysis to identify the strengths and challenges for any individual or groups of individuals. Although this book focuses on youth with lifelong conditions, there is a great deal of potential for occupational therapists to promote inclusive transition practices and resources for all youth. School environments may be the best setting for this approach, as the occupational therapist can provide consultation in a whole classroom, which may include students with disabilities, but many of the suggestions made by the therapist could be utilized by all of the students. For example, development of strong self-determination skills is important for all youth. Collaboration with other school personnel or community members, such as employers or recreation leaders, will be essential for any occupational therapist who wants to promote inclusive transition practices.

Capacity Building

Occupational therapists have the capacity to contribute to the process and outcomes of transitioning to adulthood for all youth with disabilities. Our capacity is based upon our knowledge, skills, and abilities to analyze and use occupation. Our occupational therapy lens is unique, and evidence has shown that a lens of occupation can make a difference in people's lives (Law, Steinwender, & Leclair, 1998).

The emerging evidence about transitions to adulthood suggests that PEO interactions must be addressed, and preferred outcomes identified by youth, families, and others should be at the level of participation, contribution, citizenship, and quality of life (Stewart et al., 2009). This fits well with occupation-based practice models, but it means that occupational therapists need to move away from component-based practices, which focus more on changing client factors at the level of body functions and structures. Occupational therapists working in school systems need to focus clinical reasoning efforts on identifying strategies that will directly impact an individual's participation in occupations that are meaningful to him or her now and in the future, such as engaging students in experiences that promote self-determination. School-based occupational therapists should not be addressing just component sensory, motor, or cognitive skills, but rather situating them within occupation and occupational performance to build a student's capacity for full participation in daily environments.

Evidence is supporting a strengths-based approach to services and supports. Again, client-centered and family-centered approaches foster this, but many therapists still tend to focus on the "problems" instead of the strengths of youth and their families (Stewart & Rosenbaum, 2007). Strengths-based or asset-building approaches (Kretzmann & McKnight, 1983) promote capacity building by focusing on assets rather than deficits. One simple step to take in this direction is to start any meeting or discussion about a client with a positive statement about his or her strengths. Occupational therapists can also support youth and parents to always think first about their strengths and to view asking for assistance as a sign of personal strength in knowing what they need and want.

Children with ASD present with a range of abilities, and they can demonstrate strengths that typically developing children do not have (Crabtree & DeLany, 2011), such as math and problem-solving skills. Occupational therapists working with children, such as Jenny, can build on their strengths to encourage their participation in daily classroom routines. Intervention models that promote the development of making choices and understanding social rules can promote the development of self-determination as Jenny gets older (Crabtree & Sherwin, 2011). Occupational therapists can use our unique clinical reasoning and PEO analysis to identify the developmental sequencing and steps needed at different ages and stages of life to build a young person's capacities for future occupations such as work. Within the high school setting, often the role of the occupational therapist shifts to more consultation, to work with school staff and the community at large to promote opportunities for meaningful experiences in his or her community. An occupational therapist's skills in task analysis and modifying occupations and environments are extremely useful in promoting experiential learning in naturally occurring contexts (Spencer, 2010).

Research about capacity building provides evidence to guide our own transitions in our views and practices to support inclusion and participation for all youth with disabilities. We need to move toward the following:

> An increased focus on self-determination, which has been shown to positively influence the transition process for some youth. Some examples have been described in the chapters of this book.

> A shift in focus from "independence" to "interdependence" (Gooden-Ledbetter, Cole, Maher, & Condeluci, 2007), which acknowledges that there can be mutual benefits to people sharing experiences and supporting and learning from each other in daily occupations.

> Development of peer mentorship programs and resources for youth and parents. The evidence about peer mentorship is positive (Foster & MacLeod, 2004; Grove & Giraud-Saunders, 2003) (Figure 8-5). Occupational therapists can assist individual clients who are in transition to meet up with young adults and share their experiences and lessons learned. Meetings can be in person or through social networking media. Peer mentorship programs have been shown to benefit everyone involved, including mentors, mentees, and therapists (Stewart, 2003). Occupational therapists can also be supportive of parents of youth in transition by connecting them with parent networks in the community.

> Use of community capacity-building strategies (DSD, 2009), which can be beneficial within our own community of practice, whether it is an institution, school, or region. Occupational therapists can build community capacity by meeting with people from other agencies and community services who are interested in collaborating. There is some evidence about the impact of capacity building workshops with employers and other community members to increase their understanding and capacity to offer community-based experiences and opportunities for youth with disabilities (Wynn, Stewart, Law, Burke-Gaffney, & Moning, 2007).

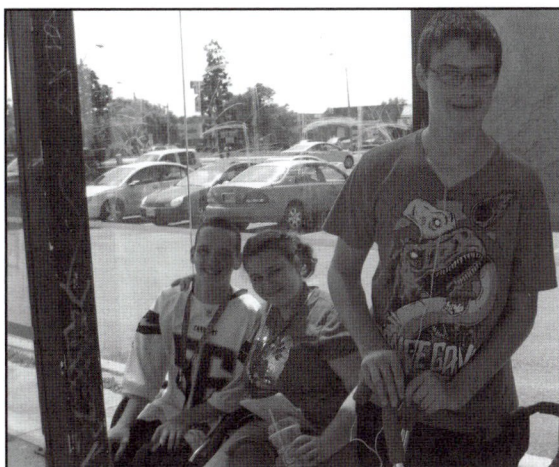

Figure 8-5. Peer mentorship can be a positive support for youth with disabilities as they begin to explore their community.

Accessible and Useful Information, Resources, and Services

Occupational therapists are well aware of the importance of informed decision making for clients. We can use some of the guidelines related to health literacy (Nielsen-Bohlman et al., 2004; Rootman & Gordeon-El-Bihbety, 2008), as described in the previous section, to provide youth with age-appropriate and understandable information about the key occupations, and changes in occupations, as they enter adulthood. Different forms of information sharing can be used, depending on the audience, such as verbal presentations, written brochures and summaries, and online resources. There are some important transition topics for occupational therapists to consider when supporting youth to develop their capacity for making their own decisions. Evidence-based recommendations for occupational therapists working with youth such as Jenny include:

» "What's ahead, what's coming?"—Information to enable youth and families to plan and prepare. Occupational therapists can use their occupational and task analysis skills to identify the steps and demands involved in future adult occupations. This information will guide youth and parents to develop realistic action plans.

» "What's out there?"—Information to increase awareness of youth and families of all options to enable their decision making about a particular direction or action plan.

» "What can I do?"—Information to promote the understanding of a youth's strengths and assets, which can assist in the development of person-centered transition plans and goals.

» "What works?"—Information that summarizes recent evidence about interventions for children and youth with ASD and about transition services and supports. This includes providing specific information about occupational therapy practice to answer the question: "What can you do for me?"

Education and Research

Education can be personal (our own professional development) or focused on other people. Occupational therapists are regulated professionals who are responsible for their own professional development. When occupational therapists make a transition to another practice area, or move into a new program, they must educate themselves about the system they will be working within and other environmental factors that could impact their practice (e.g., funding models). As more occupational therapists become involved in multidisciplinary transition teams, we must stay informed about the most recent evidence, including both research and theoretical approaches. This type of professional education can also support our efforts to advocate for more occupational therapists on transition teams. We can educate others about our knowledge and skills related to occupation and how we can help to better understand the interactions between the various domains of transition, such as education, employment, housing, and socialization.

Education is a form of service delivery that draws upon principles of learning, adult education, and communication strategies (Berger, 2009). Educational activities with clients can be informal, through demonstration or verbal discussion, or more formal, through group sessions and workshops. Occupational therapists should always consider three key elements when planning any educational activity:

1. The audience—Occupational therapists need to know enough about the client(s), family members, and others to match our communication style and content with their knowledge levels and needs.

2. The environment within which occupational therapists will be providing education—The client's home, community, institution, etc.

3. The content of our educational activities—What is the knowledge level and detail, how is it best conveyed, in what form, etc. This element includes consideration of the information we will be providing. Strategies for making information accessible were discussed in the prior section, but it is important to recognize that education is more than just giving information.

The organization of these elements should be familiar to occupational therapists, as it is another example of a PEO analysis. Effective educational strategies find the best PEO fit for each activity and situation. An analysis of PEO fit at different ages and stages of Jenny's development will assist an occupational therapist in developing useful educational strategies. In childhood, most of the education will be with parents, teachers, and other service providers, to contribute to their understanding of Jenny's abilities and challenges by adding an occupational perspective. For example, occupational therapists are often educating people in the daily environments of a child with ASD about the sensory qualities of the environment, how those affect the child, and strategies to modify the environment to enable the child to participate without experiencing sensory overload. Teachers also need to understand the role of the occupational therapist within the school setting, so they know when to call on an occupational therapist for support. As Jenny gets older and starts to take some responsibility for her own self-management, the occupational therapist will begin to educate Jenny herself, so she can begin to solve problems as they arise, learn to ask for appropriate supports when she needs them, and plan for the future.

Occupational therapists can also contribute to the ongoing development of evidence by engaging in clinical research. We can develop standard procedures for gathering data about our services and clients, and these data can be aggregated and analyzed for quality assurance and program evaluations. Occupational therapists who want to try a new intervention or strategy for children and youth with ASD, such as relationship development intervention (Gutstein & Sheely, 2002) or a circle of friends (Pallis, 2010), can conduct a critical appraisal of the research on these approaches to make a decision about using them in their own clinical practice. We can then set up a single subject or case study design to monitor the progress of a client or clients, and then review this evidence with other therapists to determine future practice. This could be an evidence-based approach for the therapist working with Jenny who wants to start using a collaborative consultation service model in the school setting. Occupational therapy departments can promote an evidence-based approach to practice as well. When a department purchases a new assessment tool or outcome measure, each therapist can be asked to administer the measure with two or three clients and submit their data after a period of time. The aggregated data can then be shared at a department meeting to facilitate a discussion about the use of this measure within the practice setting. This will be helpful in the long term for clients, such as Jenny, as it is anticipated that more assessment measures that address the participation level of functioning of youth and young adults will be available by the time she is an adolescent and young adult (Sax & Thoma, 2002).

Conclusion

Building capacity through collaboration, information, education, and research may sound simple, but the evidence about transitions to adulthood for youth with disabilities has identified multiple systems, factors, and domains that must all be considered in interaction with each other. Occupational therapists have a great deal to contribute to building the capacity of youth, families, communities, services, and systems through sharing our knowledge about PEO transactions and the analysis and application of occupations, tasks, and activities. Some of our traditional views and practices require some changes and transitions if occupational therapists want to meet the needs of our young clients with lifelong disabilities. We can also build our own capacity to provide collaborative, capacity-building occupational therapy services with youth with disabilities in their natural environments, and also expand our thinking and practices to promote inclusive environments and transition practices for all youth. We will know that our own transitions have been successful when Jenny is a young adult who is participating in occupations that are meaningful, important, and developmentally appropriate within an inclusive community and society.

Review Questions

1. What are some similar issues and challenges faced by youth with any disability?

2. Can you describe the metaphor for the BJA model and how it fits with current views on transitioning?

3. What are some current gaps in the occupational therapist's knowledge regarding evidence around transitioning to adulthood, and what are some recommendations for filling in the gaps?

4. Identify three "first steps" that an occupational therapist can take right away to make changes in practice that will benefit youth with disabilities through childhood, adolescence, and transitions to adulthood?

References

Barnes, K. J., & Turner, K. D. (2001). Team collaborative practices between teachers and occupational therapists. *American Journal of Occupational Therapy, 55*(1), 83-89.

Bazyk, S., & Case-Smith, J. (2010). School-based occupational therapy. In J. Case-Smith & J. C. O'Brien (Eds.), *Occupational therapy for children* (6th ed., pp. 713-743). St. Louis, MO: Elsevier.

Berger, S. (2009). Client education. In E. B. Crepeau, E. S. Cohn, & B. A. Boyt Schell (Eds.), *Willard and Spackman's occupational therapy* (11th ed., pp. 418-432). New York, NY: Lippincott Williams & Wilkins.

Clark, G. F. (2008). Getting into a collaborative school routine. In B. Hanft & J. Shepherd (Eds.), *Collaborating for student success: A guide for school-based occupational therapy.* Bethesda, MD: American Occupational Therapy Association Press.

Committee on Disability in America. (2007). Health care transitions for young people. In M. J. Field & A. M. Jette (Eds.), *Future of disability in America* (pp. 4-1). Washington, DC: The National Academies Press.

Crabtree, L., & DeLany, J. V. (2011). Autism: Promoting social participation and mental health. In S. Bazyk (Ed.), *Mental health promotion, prevention, and intervention with children and youth* (pp. 163-187). Bethesda, MD: American Occupational Therapy Association Press.

Crabtree, L., & Sherwin, A. B. (2011). Begin with the end in mind: Promoting mental health, social participation and self-determination in the transition from school to adult life. In S. Bazyk (Ed.), *Mental health promotion, prevention, and intervention with children and youth* (pp. 267-286). Bethesda, MD: AOTA Press.

Department for Social Development. (2009). *Voluntary and community sector community capacity building.* Northern Ireland, UK. Retrieved October 30, 2011 from www.dsdni.gov.uk/vcni-community-capacity-building.pdf

Foster, S., & MacLeod, J. (2004). The role of mentoring relationships in the career development of successful deaf persons. *Journal of Deaf Studies and Deaf Education, 9*(4), 442-458.

Gooden-Ledbetter, M. J., Cole, M. T., Maher J. K., & Condeluci, A. (2007). Self-efficacy and interdependence as predictors of life satisfaction for people with disabilities: Implications for independent living programs. *Journal of Vocational Rehabilitation, 27*(3), 153-161.

Gorter, J. W., Stewart, D., & Woodbury-Smith, M. (2011). Youth in transition: Care, health, and development. *Child: Care, Health, and Development,* 37(6), 757-763.

Grove, B., & Giraud-Saunders, A. (2003). Connecting with connexions: The role of the personal adviser with young people with special educational and support needs. *Support for Learning, 18*(1), 12-17.

Gutstein, S. E. & Sheely, R. K. (2002). *Relationship development intervention with children, adolescents and adults: Social and emotional development activities for asperger syndrome, autism, PDD, and NLD.* Philadelphia, PA: Jessica Kingsley.

Halfon, N., & Hochstein, M. (2002). Life course health development: An integrated framework for developing health, policy, and research. *Milbank Quarterly, 80*(3), 433-479. doi:10.1111/1468-0009.00019

Hamdani, Y., Jetha, A., & Norman, C. (2011). Systems thinking perspectives applied to healthcare transition for youth with disabilities: a paradigm shift for practice, policy, and research. *Child Care, Health, and Development, 37* (6), 806-814. doi: 10.1111/j.1365-2214.2011.01313.x

Hanft, B., & Shepherd, J. (Eds.) (2008). *Collaborating for student success: A guide for school-based occupational therapy.* Bethesda, MD: American Occupational Therapy Association Press.

Hawkins, M. T., Letcher, P., Sanson, A., O'Connor, M., Toumbourou, J. W., & Olsson, C. (2011). Stability and change in positive development during young adulthood. *Journal of Youth and Adolescence, 40*(11), 1436-1452.

Hines, J. T. (2008). Making collaboration work in inclusive high school classrooms: Recommendations for principals. *Intervention in School and Clinic, 43*, 277-282.

Ho., K., Bloch, R., Gondocz, T., Laprise, R., Perrier, L., Ryan, D.,...Wenghofer, E. (2004). Technology enabled-knowledge-translation: Frameworks to promote research and practice. *Journal of Continuing Education in the Health Professions, 24*(2), 70-78.

King, S., Teplicky, R., King, G., & Rosenbaum, P. (2004). Family-centred service for children with cerebral palsy and their families: A review of the literature. *Seminars in Pediatric Neurology, 11*, 78-86.

Kingsnorth, S., Gall, C., Beayni, S., & Rigby, P. (2011). Parents as transition experts? Qualitative findings from a pilot parent-led peer support group. *Child: Care, Health, and Development, 37*, 833-840.

Kretzmann, J. P., & McKnight, J. L. (1983). *Building communities from the inside out. A path toward finding and mobilizing a community's assets.* Evanston, IL: Asset-Based Community Development Institute. www.abcdinstitute.org/capacity/

Law, M. (1998). Does client-centred practice make a difference? In M. Law (Ed.), *Client-centred occupational therapy.* Thorofare, NJ: SLACK Incorporated.

Law, M., & Telford, J. (2008). Knowledge transfer strategies. In M. Law & J. MacDermid (Eds.), *Evidence-based rehabilitation: A guide to practice.* Thorofare, NJ: SLACK Incorporated.

Law, M., Steinwender, S., & Leclair, L. (1998). Occupation, health and well-being. *Canadian Journal of Occupational Therapy, 65*, 82-91.

Learning Disabilities Association of Canada (LDAC). (2007). *Putting a Canadian face on learning disabilities (PACFOLD).* Ottawa, Ontario, Canada: LDAC.

Leiter, V., & Waugh, A. (2009). Moving out: Residential independence among young adults with disabilities and the role of families. *Marriage and Family Review, 45*, 519-537.

Luecking, R. G., & Wittenburg, D. (2009). Providing supports to youth with disabilities transitioning to adulthood. Case descriptions from the Youth Transition Demonstration. *Journal of Vocational Rehabilitation, 30*, 241-251. doi 10.3233/JVR-2009-0464

MacDermid, J. (2008). Practice guidelines, algorithms, and clinical pathways. In M. Law & J. MacDermid (Eds.), *Evidence-based rehabilitation: A guide to practice.* Thorofare, NJ: SLACK Incorporated.

Mahmood, D., Dicianno, B., & Bellin, M. (2011). Self-management, preventable conditions and assessment of care among young adults with myelomeningocele. *Child: Care, Health, and Development, 37*, 861-865.

Mankey, T. (2011). Occupational therapists' beliefs and involvement with secondary transition planning. *Physical and Occupational Therapy in Pediatrics, 31*(4), 345-358.

McConachie, H. (2011). Improving mental health transitions for young people with autism spectrum disorder. *Child: Care, Health, and Development, 37*(6), 764-766. doi: 10.1111/j.1365-2214.2011.01238.x

Miller-Kuhaneck, H. (2004). *Autism: A comprehensive occupational therapy approach,* (2nd ed.). Bethesda, MD: American Occupational Therapy Association Press.

Missiuna, C., Pollock, N., Levac, D., Campbell, W. N., Whalen, S. D., Bennett, S. M.,...Russell, D. J. (2012). Partnering for change: An innovative school-based occupational therapy service delivery model for children with developmental coordination disorder. *Canadian Journal of Occupational Therapy, 79*(1), 41-50.

Nicholas, D. B., Picone, G., Vigneux, A., McCormick, K., Mantulak, A., McClure, M., MacCulloch, R. (2009). Evaluation of an online peer support network for adolescents with chronic kidney disease. *Journal of Technology in Human Services, 27*, 23-33.

Nielsen-Bohlman, L., Panzer, A. M. & Kindig, D. A. (Eds.). (2004). *Health literacy: A prescription to end confusion.* Washington, DC: National Academies Press.

Pallis, B. (2010). Circle of friends: The path to inclusion. Retrieved October 30, 2011 from www.circleofriends.org/

Priestly, M. (Ed.). (2001). *Disability and the life course. Global perspectives.* Cambridge, UK: Cambridge University Press.

Reid, D., Chiu, T., Sinclair, G., Wehrmann, S., & Naseer, Z. (2006). Outcomes of an occupational therapy school-based consultation service for students with fine motor difficulties. *Canadian Journal of Occupational Therapy, 73*, 215-224.

Repetto, J. B., Gibson, R. W., Lubbers, J., Gritz, S., & Reiss, J. (2008). A statewide study of knowledge and attitudes regarding health care transition. *Career Development for Exceptional Individuals, 31*(1), 5-13.

Rootman, I., & Gordon-El-Bihbety, D. (2008). *A vision for a health literate Canada. Report of the expert panel on health literacy.* Ottawa, Ontario, Canada: Canadian Public Health Association.

Salvatori, P., Jung B., Missiuna C., Stewart D., Law, M., & Wilkins, S. (2006). *The McMaster Lens for Occupational Therapists.* Hamilton, Ontario, Canada: McMaster University.

Sax, C. L. & Thoma, C. A. (2002). *Transition assessment: Wise practices for quality lives.* Baltimore, MD: Paul H. Brookes Publishing.

Sayers, B. R. (2008). Collaboration in school settings: A critical appraisal of the topic. *Journal of Occupational Therapy, Schools, and Early Intervention, 1*, 170-179.

Schwartz, L. S., Tuchman, L. K., Hobbie, W. L., & Ginsberg, J. P. (2011). A social-ecological model of readiness for transition to adult-oriented care for adolescents and young adults with chronic health conditions. *Child: Care, Health, and Development, 37*(6), 883-895.

Social Support Research Program. (2005). *Online support for adolescents with cerebral palsy and spina bifida. Final report.* Retrieved November 11 from www.abilityonline.org/sites/default/files/Online%20support%20youth%20 with%20CP%20and%20SB.pdf

Spencer, K. C. (2010). Transition services: From school to adult life. In J. Case-Smith & J. C. O'Brien (Eds.), *Occupational therapy for children* (6th ed., pp. 812-832). St. Louis, MO: Elsevier.

Stewart, D. (2003). Peer mentorship as an environmental support for adolescents and young adults with disabilities. In L. Letts, P. Rigby, & D. Stewart (Eds.), *Using environments to enable occupational performance.* Thorofare, NJ: SLACK Incorporated.

Stewart, D. (2009). Transition to adult services for youth with disabilities: Current evidence to guide future research. *Developmental Medicine and Child Neurology, 51* (Suppl. 4), 169-173.

Stewart D., & Rosenbaum, P. (2007). Commentary perspectives on transitions: Rethinking services for children and youth with developmental disabilities. *Archives of Physical Medicine and Rehabilitation. 88*(8), 1080-1082.

Stewart, D., Law, M., Rosenbaum, P., & Willms, D. (2001). A qualitative study of the transition to adulthood for youth with disabilities. *Physical and Occupational Therapy in Pediatrics, 21*(4), 3-22.

Stewart, D., Law, M., Young, N., Forhan, M., Healy, H., Burke-Gaffney, J., & Freeman, M. (2008). *Understanding the transitional tensions of youth with disabilities in Canada. Identifying key research gaps. Penultimate report to Human Resources Social Development Canada (HRSDC).* Hamilton, Ontario, Canada: McMaster University. Unpublished document.

Stewart, D., Freeman, M., Law, M., Healy, H., Burke-Gaffney, J., Forhan, M.,...Guenther, S. (2009). *"The best journey to adult life" for youth with disabilities. An evidence-based model and best practice guidelines for the transition to adulthood for youth with disabilities.* Hamilton, Ontario, Canada: McMaster University. Retrieved October 30, 2011 from http://transitions.canchild.ca/en/OurResearch/bestpractices.asp

Tomchek, S., & Case-Smith, J. (2009). *Occupational therapy practice guidelines for children and adolescents with autism.* Bethesda, MD: American Occupational Therapy Association Press.

Villenueve, M. (2009). A critical examination of school-based occupational therapy collaborative consultation. *Canadian Journal of Occupational Therapy, 76*, 206-218.

Wagner, M., Newman, L., Cameto, R., Levine, P., & Garza, N. (2006). *An overview of findings from wave 2 of the National Longitudinal Transition Study-2 (NLTS2).* National Center for Special Education Research. US Department of Education.

World Health Organization (WHO). (1998). *Health Promotion Glossary.* Geneva, Switzerland: WHO.

World Health Organization (WHO). (2001). *International classification of functioning, disability and health (ICF).* Geneva, Switzerland: WHO.

Wynn, K., Stewart, D., Law, M., Burke-Gaffney, J., & Moning, T. (2007) Creating connections: A community capacity building project with parents and youth with disabilities in transition to adulthood. *Physical and Occupational Therapy in Paediatrics, 26*(4), 89-103.

Financial Disclosures

Linda Armour has no financial or proprietary interest in the materials presented herein.

Kim Carey has no financial or proprietary interest in the materials presented herein.

Dr. Mary Forhan has no financial or proprietary interest in the materials presented herein.

Matt Freeman has no financial or proprietary interest in the materials presented herein.

Jan Burke-Gaffney has no financial or proprietary interest in the materials presented herein.

Grace Herron has no financial or proprietary interest in the materials presented herein.

Dr. Mary Law has no financial or proprietary interest in the materials presented herein.

Karen Margallo has no financial or proprietary interest in the materials presented herein.

Dr. Sandra Moll has no financial or proprietary interest in the materials presented herein.

Andrea Morrison has no financial or proprietary interest in the materials presented herein.

Baljit Samrai has no financial or proprietary interest in the materials presented herein.

Debra Stewart has no financial or proprietary interest in the materials presented herein.

Christy Taberner has no financial or proprietary interest in the materials presented herein.

Kevin Tregunno has no financial or proprietary interest in the materials presented herein.

Index

adaptation perspective, 35-36

adulthood, transition to. *See* transition to adulthood

Americans with Disabilities Act (ADA), 8

assessment, 40-41
    of youth living with obesity, 128-130
    of youth with cerebral palsy, 53-54
    of youth with developmental disability, 73-74
    of youth with learning disabilities, 89-99
    of youth with mental illness, 109-114

Assessment of Life Habits (LIFE-H), 33

assistive devices, 80-81
    dynamic assessment of use of, 93-95
    for youth with learning disabilities, 77-101

Assistive Technology Act of 1998, 80

attention deficit disorder (ADD), 77-101

Autism Act (UK), 8-9

autism spectrum disorder (ASD), 135, 138, 142-143, 145, 146

barriers, 13

Best Journey to Adult Life (BJA) model, 137, 138

Canadian Model of Occupational Performance (CMOP), 29-30
    occupational categories in, 31-32

Canadian Occupational Performance Measure (COPM), 33, 49-50
    for youth living with obesity, 126-127
    post-intervention scores in, 64
    for youth with learning disability, 81, 87-89, 100

cerebral palsy, transition to independent living with, 47-65

Charter of Rights and Freedoms (Canada), 8

Children's Assessment of Participation and Enjoyment (CAPE), 33

Circle of Friends, 68

co-op placements, 69-70

cognitive-neurological performance
    in independent living arrangements, 52
    of youth with Down syndrome, 72
    of youth with learning disability, 89-95

collaborative consultation model, 30, 78, 143-145

community
    accessibility issues in, 56
    information, resources, and services of, 140-141
    resources for youth living with obesity in, 130-133
    support systems of, 8, 137-138
    work experience in, 67-75

community capacity-building
    principles of, 139-140
    strategies for, 146

Comprehensive Test of Phonological Processing, 86

computers, as assistive devices, 80-81

conceptual models, 27

craniopharyngioma, obesity and, 123-134

cultural environment, 51-52
    evidence about, 6, 7-9
    for youth with Down syndrome, 72

Dells-Kaplan Executive Function System, 86

development
    with developmental disability, 69-70
    with learning disability, 78-79
    in McMaster Lens for Occupational Therapists, 35-36
    with mental illness, 106-108
    need for research on, 136
    with obesity, 124-126
    theories and models about, 16-17
    in transition to independent living, 48-50

developmental transitions
    in youth with disabilities, 1-21
    in youth with mental health issues, 103-119

disability. *See also* learning disability; physical disability; *specific conditions*
    areas of challenges of, 135-136
    attitudes toward, 13
    developmental, 67-75
    theories and models of, 17-18
    WHO definition of, 18

Disability Creation Process, 18

domains, 9-12

Down syndrome, work experience for youth with, 67-75

dynamics of doing, 78

education
domain of, 11
in knowledge development, 141-142
of occupational therapists, 147-149
post-secondary, for youth with learning disabilities, 77-101

embodied marginalization, 13

emerging adulthood, 17

employment domain, 11. *See also* work

enablement skill, 73

environmental approach, 37-43, 53-54, 56-58, 72-73

environmental factors
for youth living with obesity, 127
in transition to post-secondary education, 88
in youth with cerebral palsy, 51-52
in youth with Down syndrome, 71-72
in youth with physical disabilities, 51-52

event markers, xiv

Goal Attainment Scaling (GAS), 33

goals
of individual direct therapy, 55-58
prioritizing, 54
review of, 63-64
vision for future and, 50

government supports, 8

group-based interventions. *See* interventions, group-based

Hamilton Family Network, 68

handwriting skills, 91-93, 99-100

health conditions, complex, obesity and, 123-134

health literacy, definitions of, 140

health trajectories, 17

hearing assessment, 89

high school work experience program, 68

holistic approaches, 136

impairment/conditions, types of, 4-5

independent living
arrangements in, 61
definition of, 48
transitions to, 47-65

independent living skills program
format and content of, 59-63
goals in, 65
participant criteria and program focus of, 58-59
sample schedule for, 62-63

Individuals with Disabilities Education Improvement Act (IDEA), 9, 138

information, accessibility and usefulness of, 140-141, 147

institutional environment, 6

interdependence
concept of, 48
focus on, 146

International Classification of Functioning, Disability and Health (ICF), 18

Internet-based information, 140-141

interprofessional collaboration, 145

interventions. *See also* McMaster Lens for Occupational Therapists approach; therapeutic approaches; *specific approaches*
group-based
developing and planning, 59
goals in, 65
independent living skills program in, 60-61
for youth with cerebral palsy, 58
individual direct
for youth with cerebral palsy, 55-58
for youth with Down syndrome, 73
for youth with mental illness, 114-117

Job Connect, 105

job search skills, 55-56

job skills, 72, 73

journal writing, 131

keyboarding skills, 93-95

knowledge development, 141-142

knowledge gap, 142

learning disability
assistive technology for, 80-81
assistive technology for youth with, 77-101
definition of, 79-80
diagnosis of, 80
education transition planning for, 11
occupational therapy recommendations for, 96-98

legislation, 136. *See also specific laws*
on adult transitions, 10

for collaborative transition planning, 137-138

impact of, 8-9

on rights, employment, and rehabilitation, 10

leisure, 31-32, 52

Leisure Interest Inventory, 128, 129

leisure pursuits, obesity and, 123-134

lifecourse perspective, 16-17, 35

living arrangements, 11-12. *See also* independent living

McMaster Lens for Occupational Therapists approach, 28-44

    assessment component of, 40-41, 53-54, 73-74

    development component of, 35-36

    development of, 29-30

    fine tuning, 41-42

    occupation component of, 31-33

    outcome component of, 43-44

    Person-Environment-Occupation component of, 36-37

    practice scenarios of, 31

    spirituality component of, 34

    theoretical component of, 37-40

    in transitions to independent living, 47-65

    treatment component of, 42-43

    for youth living with obesity

        assessment in, 128-130

        fine tuning, 130

        intervention in, 130-131

        occupation, spirituality, and development components of, 124-126

        outcomes for, 131-134

        PEO analysis and theoretical approaches in, 126-128

    for youth with developmental disabilities

        outcomes in, 75

        PEO analysis in, 70-72

        treatment approaches in, 73-74

        work experience program in, 69-75

    for youth with learning disabilities, 77-101

        assessment and intervention in, 89-99

        occupation, spirituality, and development in, 78-79

        PEO analysis in, 81-8 9

        theoretical approaches in, 81-89

    for youth with mental illness, 106, 119

        assessment in, 109-114

        intervention strategies in, 114-117

        occupation, spirituality, and development components of, 106-108

        outcomes in, 117-119

        PEO analysis and theoretical approaches in, 108-109

        theoretical approaches in, 108-109

    for youth with physical disabilities

        fine tuning, 54

        occupation, spirituality, and development in, 69-70

        outcomes of, 63-64

        PEO analysis in, 50-52

        theoretical approaches in, 52-55

        therapeutic approaches in, 55-64

        treatment component of, 54-55

McMaster University, occupational therapy program of, 27-44. *See also* McMaster Lens for Occupational Therapists approach

meal planning/preparation

    developing skills for, 56-57

    goals for, 61

Meaningful Lives, 119

mental health issues, employment and, 103-119

mental illness

    education and employment prospects with, 107

    functional issues in, 115-116

    physical, cognitive, emotional, and social limitations in, 114

mind mapping software, 95

mobility, 51

Motor-Free Visual Perception Test (MVPT-3), 89, 91

motor function, 89

Nagi model, 18

Networks of Support, 68

No Child Left Behind Act, 9

obesity

    beliefs about and attitudes toward, 124, 125

    bullying and, 124

    self-esteem and, 124, 130-131

    socialization and leisure pursuits with, 123-134

occupation

    categories of, 31-32

    theories and models of, 18-19, 27

occupational analysis, 9-12

    in McMaster Lens for Occupational Therapists, 31-33

meaningful, 31-32
  for youth living with obesity, 124-126, 127-128, 133
  social and community life domain of, 12
  in transition to independent living, 48-50
  in transition to post-secondary education, 89
  for youth with developmental disability, 69-70
  for youth with Down syndrome, 72
  for youth with learning disability, 78-79
  for youth with mental illness, 106-108
occupational performance and engagement, 19
Occupational Performance History Interview II (OPHI-II), 33
occupational therapists
  capacity building in, 145-146
  clinical research of, 148-149
  education of, 147-148
  transitions for, 142-149
occupational therapy
  evidence about, 14-16
  models of, 18-19, 27
  theories of, 27-44
outcomes, 43-44
  evaluation of, 63-64
  identification and measurement of, 14
  for youth living with obesity, 131-134
  participation-level measures of, 136
  for youth with cerebral palsy, 63-64
  for youth with Down syndrome, 75
  for youth with mental illness, 117-119

parents' home, transitions from, 47-65
peer mentorship programs, 146, 147
PEO (person-environment-occupation) analysis
  in transition to post-secondary education, 81-89
  in youth living with obesity, 126-128
  in youth with cerebral palsy, 50-52
  in youth with developmental disability, 70-72
  in youth with learning disability, 88-89
PEO (person-environment-occupation) interactions, 12-13
PEO (person-environment-occupation) Model
  for transition, 15, 19, 20, 30, 36-37, 136
  in McMaster occupational Lens theory, 30

person factors
  of youth living with obesity, 126-127
  of youth with cerebral palsy, 50-51
  of youth with Down syndrome, 71
  of youth with learning disabilities, 88
personal digital assistants, 95
personal risk factors/barriers, 4-5
personal supports/facilitators, 3-4
physical disabilities, independent living with, 47-66
physical environment, 51
  evidence about, 5, 6
  in work experience of youth with Down syndrome, 71
physical function assessment, 89-93
policy impact, 8
positive development, 17
practice guidelines, 137
  collaborative, 137-139
productivity, 31-32, 52
  learning disability and, 87
psychiatric disorders, education transition planning for, 11
psychoeducational assessment, 81-87
  functional implications of, 87
  key areas of, 82
  for youth with learning disability, 81-87
psychoemotional approach, 52, 108-109, 129-130
psychosis, employment prospects and, 103-107
psychosocial rehabilitation, 109
public transportation
  access to, 55
  planning use of, 61

Rehabilitation Act, Section 504, 9
research, xv
  in knowledge development, 141-142
  occupational therapy, 147-149
  on transition to adulthood, 1-21
residential independence, 49
resources, accessibility of, 140-141, 147
Rosenberg Self-Esteem Scale, 130

schizophrenia, work transition for youth with, 103-119
school-based collaborative consultation, 143-144
School Function Assessment (SFA), 33

school-related occupations, 78
school-work transition, 11
self-care, 31-32, 52
self-determination, 3-4, 146
self-esteem, obesity and, 124, 130-131
services/systems
    accessible and useful, 140-141, 147
    culture of, 8-9
    future directions for, 137
    person-environment interactions in, 13
    research on, 137-138
SMART objectives, 54
social and community life domain, 12
social environment, 5-7, 51
    for youth with Down syndrome, 72
social interaction/network
    for youth living with obesity, 125-126, 127,
        129, 131, 133
    online, 140-141
socialization, obesity and, 123-134
sociocultural approach, 52-54, 72, 127, 130
sociocultural factors, 30, 38-42
Special Educational Needs Code of Practice
    (UK), 9
speech recognition software, 94
spirituality
    in McMaster Lens for Occupational
        Therapists, 34
    in transition to independent living, 48-50
    in youth living with obesity, 124-126
    in youth with developmental disability,
        69-70
    in youth with learning disability, 78-79
    in youth with mental illness, 106-108
support, versus barriers, 13
support systems
    collaborative, 137-139
    community level, 138-139
    future directions for, 137
    for youth with Down syndrome, 68
supported employment
    assessment approaches in, 112-114
    effectiveness of, 111
    intervention strategies in, 114-117
    occupational therapists providing, 111-112
    outcomes of, 117-119
    principles of, 109-111

task adaptation, 56-57
temporal environment, 6

temporary work, 105
text scanning/reading software, 95
theoretical approaches
    categories of, 38-39
    in McMaster Lens for Occupational
        Therapists, 37-40
    in transition to post-secondary education,
        81-89
    treatment consistent with, 42
    to youth living with obesity, 126-128
    to youth with cerebral palsy, 52-55
    to youth with developmental disability, 72
therapeutic approaches
    group-based, 58
    individual, 55-58
    of McMaster Lens for Occupational
        Therapists, 42-43
    outcomes for, 63-64
    in transition to post-secondary education,
        89-99
    to youth living with obesity, 130-131
    to youth with developmental disability,
        73-74
Ticket to Work and Work Incentive
    Improvement Act, 9
transfer routines, safe, 58
transition services, 136
transitions to adulthood, 1-21
    collaborative initiatives and policies for,
        137-139
    complexity of, 12-13
    current knowledge about, 135-136
    environment components of, 5-9
    future research and practice directions in,
        135-149
    knowledge gaps in, 136-142
    occupation components of, 9-12
    occupational therapists' role in, 142-149
    occupational therapy for, 14-15
    person components of, 3-5
    person-environment-occupation interac-
        tions of, 12-14
    research on, 2-3
        critique of, 16-19

virtual environment, 6
vision assessment, in learning disabilities, 89
visual-motor integration (VMI), 90
visual perception, 90
visual thinking and learning software, 95

Wechsler Adult Intelligence Scales, 4th edition, 82-84
Wechsler Individual Achievement Test-III, 85
weight loss goal, 125, 133
wheelchair accessibility, 51
Wide Range Assessment of Memory & Learning, 2nd edition, 84
word prediction software, 94
work
early, impact of on teens' mental health, 107
in high school, 68, 69
in recovery from mental illness, 104-106
supported, 111-119
transitions to with mental health issues, 103-119
work accommodation process, 115-117
work environment scale, 114